Handbook
for the
Care of Infants, Toddlers,
and Young Children
with Disabilities
and Chronic Conditions

edited by   **Marilyn J. Krajicek**
Geraldine Steinke
Dalice L. Hertzberg
Nicholas Anastasiow
Susan Sandall

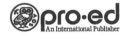

D0888307

pro·ed
An International Publisher

8700 Shoal Creek Boulevard
Austin, Texas 78757-6897

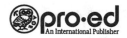

© 1997, 1996 by PRO-ED, Inc.
8700 Shoal Creek Boulevard
Austin, Texas 78757-6897

Library of Congress Cataloging-in-Publication Data

Handbook for the care of infants, toddlers, and young children with
  disabilities and chronic conditions / edited by Virginia Torrey . . .
  [et al.].
    p. cm.
  Includes bibliographical references and index.
  ISBN 0-89079-70-0 (alk. paper)
    1. Handicapped children—Care. 2. Chronically ill children—Care.
  3. Child development deviations. 4. Chronic diseases in children.
  I. Torrey, Virginia.
RJ135.H455 1997
618.92—dc21   96-49479
                                                                                      CIP

Production Manager: Alan Grimes
Production Coordinator: Karen Swain
Managing Editor: Tracy Sergo
Art Director: Thomas Barkley
Reprints Buyer: Alicia Woods
Editor: Margaret Nardecchia
Editorial Assistant: Claudette Landry
Editorial Assistant: Suzi Hunn

Printed in the United States of America

2   3   4   5   6   7   8   9   10   01   00   99   98

ACKNOWLEDGEMENTS

Marilyn J. Krajicek, EdD, RN, FAAN
Associate Professor
University of Colorado Health Sciences Center
School of Nursing
Denver, CO

Geraldine Steinke, PhD
Research Associate
University of Colorado Health Sciences Center
School of Nursing
Denver, CO

Dalice L. Hertzberg, MSN, RN, CRRN
Instructor
University of Colorado Health Sciences Center
School of Nursing
Denver, CO

Nicholas Anastasiow, PhD
Thomas Hunter Professor
Department of Special Education
Hunter College
New York, NY

Susan Sandall, PhD
Research Coordinator
The Experimental Education Unit
University of Washington
Seattle, WA

Other contributors include:

Marcia H. Bakemeyer, OTR, BNBAS, CIMI
Lynn Baumeister, MS, RN, CPNP
Joanne R. Blum, MA
Donna M. Burgess, PhD
Jennifer Munns Burnham, BS
Elizabeth Cassidy, MA
Audrey Costello, LCSW
Ann Cotton, MA, PT
Anne Davidson-Mundt, MS, RN, CPNP
Candy S. Enix, MS, CCC/SLP
Kay Alicyn Ferrell, PhD
Sara J. Fidanza, MS, RN, CNSN, PNP
Suzy Fletcher, DNS
Linda L. Frederick, BA
Jane E. Freeman BSN, RN, MS, CPNP

Margaret S. Friedman, PsyD
Edward Goldson, MD, FAAP
J. Greeley, MEd
Dan R. Griffith, PhD
Mary I. Hagedorn, PhD, RN, CNS, CPNP
Carolyn L. Hayes, RN, BSN, BS, CCM
Beverly A. Isman, RDH, MPH
Robin K. Koons, PhD
Carole Logan Kuhns, PhD, RN
Sandra K. Larson, PhD
Monte Leidholm, RRT
Marjorie Long, JD
M. Colleen LumLung, MSN, RN, CPNP
Michele M. M. Mazzocco, MEd, PhD
Diane Meckstroth, PT
Carla M. Mestas, MA
Carol Ann Moore, EdD
Ann Mullen, MSN, RN
Donna L. Nimec, MD
Ann Nord, MA, RN
Jerry L. Northern, PhD
Karen O'Keeffe, MS, RN, CPNP
Sandra Panetta, EdD
Ginette A. Pepper, PhD, RN
Carol Salbenblatt, RN, MS
Joseph Schiappacasse
Rosemary A. Simkins, MN, RN
Janet L. Speirer, BSE, MA-ECSE
Susan B. Teige, LCSW
Jay Tinglum, MA
Jodi A. Wild, BSN, RN
G. Gordon Williamson, PhD, OTR

The editors with to express thanks to the contributors who have shared their knowledge and experience in the care of infants, toddlers, and young children with disabilities and chronic conditions and their families. Our special appreciation is extended to the parents and children who work with us in developing training for caregivers and to Dr. Susan Sandall who provides support as contributor and advisor to the First Start curriculum development. We also wish to acknowledge the text design, lay-out and formatting work of Eileen Rollo, the editorial review of Carolyn Acheson, the cover design and illustrations of Kathleen Duran, and the assistance of Virginia Torrey.

INTRODUCTION

Today, child caregivers and preschool personnel are caring for children who have disabilities and chronic health conditions. This reality resulted from medical and health advances that increased survival rates for many infants with life-threatening conditions and permitted surviving children to live in their home communities. Inclusion enables children with disabilities and chronic health conditions to participate with their peers in community life, including child care and preschool.

The challenge is to see the child first as a child. For example, a child with a mild asthma condition may participate fully in every activity in your center, requiring you only to be aware of the possibility of an asthma attack and what to do in case of an attack. In contrast, other children will require modifications of the physical setting, alternative means of communicating, special feeding and positioning skills, or more physical care.

The Handbook is offered by the First Start Program to help early childhood personnel to see the child before the disability. The approach is straightforward: The child needs your warmth and competence, and you require knowledge to meet the child's special needs.

To this end, First Start faculty and consultants — in child care, health, education, and early intervention — acquaint you with chronic conditions and illnesses you may encounter in your setting. The Handbook is organized into related Parts: *Human Development, Chronic Conditions, Care Needs,* and *Communication and Community Support.* Major conditions are explained, followed by descriptions of related special needs and guidance toward achieving best-practice recommendations for meeting these needs.

In this Handbook:

- *caregivers* refers to child care workers or preschool teachers;

- *parents/guardians* refers to the adults who have legal responsibility for the child's well-being; and

- *health professionals* refers to physicians, nurses, and speech, physical, occupational and other therapists.

Because medication errors pose serious risks to children, state laws and regulations detail who can administer medications and how these people should be trained and supervised. Many repetitions of a footnote concerning administration of medication appear throughout the Handbook to stress the importance of complying with your state's requirements for this issue. Similarly, a number of other procedures (catheterization, oxygen therapy, tracheostomy care, and gastrostomy care) are subject to state regulation. If you serve a child with one of these needs, you must be trained by a licensed health care provider in the specific techniques required for safe and legal care of the individual child in accordance with the laws of your state.

In addition to providing an introduction to many conditions, this Handbook will be a ready reference. It will not be the sole resource you will need. We urge you to seek more information by reaching out — to parents, health professionals caring for the children, co-workers and supervisors, and resources in your community.

You will make a difference in the lives of the children you serve.

> *By sharing your light of love, your love of learning, and your respect for all human beings, you too can be remembered as a teacher who brought light to the darkness. What a noble achievement for one's life!*[1]

---

[1] From "Bringing Light to the Darkness: A Tribute to Teachers," by Karen Stephens, *Young Children, 49*(2), 44-46.

CONTENTS

I. Human Development

II. Chronic Conditions

III. Care Needs

IV. Communication and Community Support

Supplement: Invasive Procedures

Glossary

I. HUMAN DEVELOPMENT

Human Development: Implications

Foundations of Early Learning

Social and Emotional Development

Speech and Language Development

HUMAN DEVELOPMENT: IMPLICATIONS

I. Definitions

    A.   *Development:* the natural progression from a less complex to a more complex stage, including the biologic, intellectual, behavioral, and social skills domains.

    B.   *Growth:* the increase in size of all or part of a living being in the process of development.

    C.   *Maturation:* achievement of full growth or development.

II. Nature of development

    A.   Individual children vary in the rate and exact timing of development, but the order of developmental tasks is the same for all children.

    B.   Some variations in timing are normal, whether a disability is or is not present. Extreme variations from the normal range may indicate delays and possible disability.

III. Factors influencing development

    A.   All human development is controlled by genetics but also is influenced strongly by environment. Heredity sets the limits upon possible responses the individual may make to the environments.

    B.   Each child responds to the environment in a unique way.

    C.   Heredity and the environment interact to influence a person's development throughout the lifespan.

IV. Role of the brain

    A.   Development of the brain

        1.   The brain is only partially mature at birth and continues to develop until adulthood.

        2.   The young brain is influenced strongly by environment.

        3.   There are critical periods when the child is ready physiologically to achieve major developmental milestones (in movement and coordination, speech

and language, and cognitive development) (see Table 1). If the child is deprived of adequate stimulation during these periods, later achievement of milestones will be more difficult. A child may be deprived of stimulation, for example, if he/she has few books and toys or an undetected hearing impairment.

Table 1
Brain Maturation Periods

Critical Period	Developmental Milestones
0-2 months	Gross motor activity Immature vision and hearing Reflexes: sucking, crying, thrashing
2-3 months	More mature vision and hearing Social smile Babbling and comfort sounds
7-9 months	Mature vision and hearing Fear of strangers One-word sentences (ma-ma, pa-pa, da-da)
18-22 months	Two-word sentences "NO" First form of logic
5-7 years	Full development of hearing Guilt and responsibility School-related reasoning
9-11 years	Abstract reasoning Compassion Sexuality

Used by permission of N. Anastasiow, Department of Special Education, Hunter College of the City, University of New York.

B. Organization of the brain

   1. Each of the senses (vision, hearing, taste and smell) has its own location in the brain, and each cognitive area is organized separately. If one area is damaged, others may not be affected.

   2. There are separate cognitive areas for verbal/linguistic, music, math, spatial/visual, bodily/kinesthetic, and social capabilities. For development to occur, each cognitive area must be stimulated by the environment.

3.   Deficits may be the result of a lack of experiences rather than a disability.

V.   **Development of body systems**

A.   All sensory systems are partially mature at birth and develop rapidly after birth.

1.   Motor and visual systems have the strongest influence on learning before 7-9 months. After that point, the auditory system has more influence.

2.   Senses of smell and taste are mature in infancy, but little is known about their involvement in learning.

B.   The cognitive system may not mature until age 16-17 (with some final maturation as late as age 33).

C.   Fixed behavior patterns

1.   Reflexes (involuntary reactions to stimulation) are part of a larger set of fixed behavior patterns and aid in survival, especially in infancy (see Table 2).

a.   The lack of a reflex is a sign of neurological malfunctioning or damage.
b.   Reflexes appear in a fairly regular order and disappear according to a set time schedule, unless strengthened through experience.

2.   Emotions are another part of the set of fixed behavior patterns.

a.   Infants are emotional beings.
b.   Interactions between the child and those who provide care of the child strongly influence development.

VI.   **Periods of development**

A.   The way children understand the world and their ability to interact with the environment change dramatically as they develop.   Major changes usually are observed at the following ages:

1.   2-3 months

2.   7-9 months

Table 2
Infant Reflexes

Reflex	Description	Normal Age of Disappearance
Blinking	Infant will blink at sudden appearance of a bright light or an object near the cornea.	Lifetime reflex
Sucking	When something is placed in infant's mouth, he/she starts strong sucking movements. Sometimes sucks for stimulation during sleep.	12 months
Gag	Stimulation of back of tongue and throat should cause infant to gag.	Lifetime reflex
Rooting	Stroking cheek alongside mouth causes infant to turn toward the side and begin to suck.	4 months (awake) 12 months (asleep)
Extrusion	When tongue is depressed, infant responds by pushing it outward.	4 months
Palmar grasp (hand)	Touching palms of hands near base of fingers causes infant to clench fist.	4 months
Plantar grasp (foot)	Touching soles of feet near base of toes causes toes to curl under.	12 months
Babinski	Stroking sole of foot upward from heel on outer side and across ball of the foot causes big toe to bend up and all toes to fan out.	12 months
Moro	Sudden jarring or "drop" in elevation causes flaring of arms and legs and fanning of fingers with thumb and index finger forming a "c" shape, followed by pulling in of arms to a fetal position. Infant may cry.	4 months

continued

Table 2 (con't.)

Reflex	Description	Normal Age of Disappearance
Startle	Sudden loud noise causes flaring of arms; hands remain clenched.	4 months
Tonic neck	When infant's head is turned to one side, arm and leg extend on that side and opposite arm and leg draw to body.	6 months
Stepping	When infant is held erect with sole of foot on hard surface, he/she will simulate walking movements.	4 months

3.　18-22 months

4.　3 years

5.　4 years

6.　5-7 years

B.　Early childhood (3-5 years) is a period of rapid development of language, cognition (thinking), and emotional control.

C.　By age 3 most children have learned:

1.　Autonomy (desire to do many things by themselves) and competence (ability to do so).

2.　The family rules by which to operate.

D.　During early childhood

1.　Through their exploration of the environment, children develop ideas of how things work.

2.　The peer group becomes an important source of interaction and learning.

E.　Culture influences every developmental area as the child matures (language we speak, sense of morality, meaning of events).

F.   Premature infants

   1.   The progress of a premature infant should be measured differently than the progress of a full-term baby.

   2.   When referring to developmental scales, the preemie's *gestational age* (age since conception rather than birth) should be considered.

VII.   Developmental perspective on disability and chronic illness

A.   The environmental circumstances that foster normal development also foster the development of children with special needs. In addition, children with disabilities require therapies, training, and/or prostheses (replacements for damaged or missing parts).

B.   An impairment does not necessarily prevent development, but the rate of development of children with special needs may be slower.

VIII.   Special care needs for children with disabilities

A.   A warm, *responsive environment* encourages development and may lessen the impact of illness or disability. A negative environment increases risks and magnifies deficits.

B.   Because the young brain is more adaptable than the mature brain, *early intervention* will have more impact on development than later intervention.

   1.   When brain damage is present, another part of an infant's or child's brain may take over the tasks of the damaged area, allowing the function of the damaged area to recover.

   2.   Corrective measures for sensory impairments (such as vision and hearing impairments) should begin as early as possible because sensory systems mature so quickly.

   3.   Intellectual development of a child with cognitive delays will be greater if intervention begins early and continues throughout childhood.

   4.   A physical disability that interferes with the child's exploration of the world can be offset with early intervention.

5. Premature and low birth weight infants may be less responsive to human interaction and may be easily overstimulated but may reach normal levels of functioning in a supportive, responsive environment.

BIBLIOGRAPHY

Anastasiow, N. J. (1986). *Development and disability.* Baltimore: Paul H. Brookes.

Brazelton, T. B. (1992). *Touchpoints: Your child's emotional and behavioral development.* New York: Addison-Wesley.

Gormly, A. V., & Brodzinsky, D. M. (1993). *Lifespan human development* (5th ed.). Orlando, FL: Harcourt Brace Jovanovich College Publishers.

RESOURCES

National Association for the Education of Young Children: 1-800-424-2460 or (202) 232-8777

FOUNDATIONS OF EARLY LEARNING

I. General principles

A. Theorists explain learning from different points of view including

   1. the unfolding of genetic programming,

   2. experiences in the environment, and

   3. interaction of genetics and the environment (the most widely accepted view).

B. Children learn best when their basic needs are met and they feel safe and secure.

C. Learning takes place in a variety of areas including cognition, language, motor, social, and emotional domains.

II. How young children learn

A. Children's interests and their need to make sense of their world motivate learning, in which they have an active role.

B. Children learn by using all their senses: seeing, hearing, tasting, smelling, touching.

C. Children learn by manipulating objects and seeing what happens.

D. Children learn from exploring their environment.

E. Developing various motor skills gives the child new ways to explore the environment and, thus, expands learning. For example:

   1. When infants develop the ability to grasp objects and to reach for objects, they learn about relationships of objects in space and increase their ability to explore objects.

   2. By walking, the child frees the hands, which in turn speeds up the child's exploration of the environment, leading to cognitive growth.

F.   Children learn through play.

1.   Through play children practice and consolidate skills they learned previously. Young children learn by doing things, exploring, touching, feeling, seeing, hearing, smelling, tasting things in the environment, and by practicing new skills.

2.   Make-believe symbolic play has a crucial role in the development of abstract thought.

G.   Young children learn by interacting socially with other children.

H.   Interaction with adults allows for learning.

1.   Young children learn basic values and language from seeing and hearing what adults around them do and say.

2.   Children acquire a sense of competence or mastery from contacts with adults around them and from dealing with toys and natural objects (concrete objects) in their environment.

I.   Children learn by repetition, by repeating an activity again and again.

J.   Development and learning vary from child to child.

1.   Different children learn at different rates.

2.   Children may learn more quickly in some areas than in others.

3.   Children vary in the ways they learn.

III. Strategies that facilitate learning in *all* children

A.   Provide a safe, secure environment that meets children's physiological needs so they are free to invest all their energy in the task of learning.

B.   Encourage children to explore the environment.

C.   Provide a rich variety of materials and activities, appropriate for all the developmental stages represented in the center.

D.   Use language to expand upon a child's utterances and actions.

E.   Use modeling; show the child *how*.

F.   Provide a learning environment that stimulates all the senses. When children see, hear, smell, taste, and touch things, they learn more and learn faster.

G.   Allow for repetition of activities; let children practice newly learned skills.

H.   Encourage interactions with other children.

IV.   **Implications for children with disabilities and special needs**

A.   Although the strategics that facilitate learning in all children apply to the learning of children with disabilities and chronic conditions, some children with special needs:

1.   May need more opportunities and practice.

2.   May need to have activities or toys adapted to their specific needs.

3.   May benefit from having behaviors or tasks broken down into smaller steps.

4.   May not reach developmental milestones in the "typical" way. For example:

   a.   A child with a hearing impairment may say his/her first word using sign language.

   b.   A child may not learn to walk but may learn to be mobile using a wheelchair.

5.   May need more time to complete an activity or a task.

6.   May have a greater need to use more of their senses in learning (multisensory approach).

B.   Some children may need help to be able to explore their environment. If so:

1.   Help children become aware of people, things, and toys in their environment.

2.   Adapt the environment as needed so the child can use intact senses.

3.   Observe and respond to the child's attempts to explore.

C.   Some children may need help to play with toys or other learning materials. Caregivers may need to:

1.   Teach basic movements (such as reaching or pushing) if needed.

2.   Help children manipulate and play with toys for longer periods of time.

D.   Some children may not have had "typical" experiences in their communities, such as frequently going to the grocery store, park, library, and so on.

E.   Field trips are particularly important.

1.   The family should be involved in planning and going on field trips.

2.   Additional appropriate activities to learn from the trip include taking photographs and making a book of the trip.

F.   Some children show uneven development across domains.

1.   Delay or impairment in one area may interfere with development or learning in another area.

2.   Delay or impairment in one area may interfere with expression or demonstration of what the child knows.

3.   Activities should be individualized to fit the child's strengths and weaknesses.

G.   Some children regress; they attain a skill, then lose it and have to re-learn the skill.

1.   The instructor should go back and re-teach the skill.

2.   The instructor should allow additional opportunities for the child to practice new skills.

H.   Some children require more structure to enable them to participate in activities.

V.   Using a developmental checklist

A.   A developmental checklist can be useful for observing and planning; it provides a framework to guide observations. It can be used to:

1.   Identify current abilities.

2.   Document a child's progress.

B.   A developmental checklist often is organized by developmental *domain* (cognitive development, language development, motor development, and so on) and the usual *sequence* of development.

BIBLIOGRAPHY

Allen, K. E., & Marotz, L. (1994). *Developmental profiles: Pre-birth through eight* (2d ed.). Albany, NY: Delmar.

Bredekamp, S. (Ed.). (1987). *Developmentally appropriate practice in early childhood programs serving children from birth through age 8.* Washington, DC: National Association for the Education of Young Children.

Furuno, S., O'Reilly, K., Hosaka, C., Inatuska, T., Aleman, T., & Zeisloft, B. (1979). *Hawaii early learning profile (HELP).* Palo Alto, CA: Vort Corp.

Glover, M. E., Preminger, J. L., & Sanford, A. R. (1988). *The early learning accomplishment profile for young children.* Winston-Salem, NC: Kaplan School Supply.

Gullo, D. (1992). *Developmentally appropriate practice teaching in early childhood.* Washington, DC: National Association of Education.

Harel, S., & Anastasiow, N. (1986). *The at-risk infant.* Baltimore: Paul H. Brookes.

Johnson-Martin, N., Attermeier, S. M., & Hacker, B. J. (1990). *The Carolina curriculum for preschoolers with special needs.* Baltimore: Paul H. Brookes.

Johnson-Martin, N., Jens, K. G., Attermeier, S. M., & Hacker, B. J. (1991). *The Carolina curriculum for infants and toddlers with special needs.* Baltimore: Paul H. Brookes.

Linder, T. W. (1993). *Transdisciplinary play-based assessment: A functional approach to working with young children* (rev.). Baltimore: Paul H. Brookes.

Schickedanz, J. A., Schickedanz, D. I., Hansen, K., & Forsyth, P. D. (1993). *Understanding children.* Mountain View, CA: Mayfield Publishing Co.

Sanford, A. R., & Zelman, J. G. (1994). *Learning accomplishment profile* (revised edition). Winston-Salem, NC: Kaplan School Supply.

Shearer, D. E., Billingsley, J., Froman, A., Hilliard, J., Johnson, F., & Shearer, M. (1994). *Portage guide to early education* (rev.). Portage, WI: Portage Project.

SOCIAL AND EMOTIONAL DEVELOPMENT

I. **Infants' social-emotional development**

   A. Infants are born with a variety of abilities that enable them to participate in early social exchanges with a responsive parent/guardian or caregiver.

      1. The newborn's cry is an inborn ability to signal needs.

         a. Babies cry whenever their nervous system is overly excited, from hunger, cold, pain, or too much stimulation.
         b. A young baby's cry is not intentional. Babies do *not* cry to "get their own way." The infant cry is involuntary.
         c. Over time, as caring adults respond to babies' cries, the babies learn that their needs will be met.

      2. Newborns, by nature, are attracted to social stimuli.

         a. Newborns are naturally attracted to faces. When parents/guardians or caregivers hold their head about 8 inches (the distance at which babies can best focus on objects) from the baby's face when interacting or feeding, they encourage the baby to look at that face.
         b. Newborns are predisposed to respond to human speech. Babies can hear quite well, and they have built-in coordination between their hearing and head movements. This causes them to turn in the direction of a voice and look at the face of the person who is speaking.

      3. Newborns have a built-in tendency to adapt to the kind of care they receive. A responsive adult fosters the baby's ability to fall into regular patterns of sleeping, waking, feeding, and eliminating.

   B. Temperament

      1. This term describes biologically based, inborn individual differences that affect how infants react and adjust to changes in their environment.

2.   Infants display temperament traits from birth. For example, some babies are active, kicking their legs and waving their arms much of the time, and other babies are much more quiet and still.

3.   Temperament traits include:

a.   *Activity level.* The amount of physical activity a child displays.

b.   *Rhythmicity.* The regularity of biological functions such as eating and sleeping.

c.   *Approach-withdrawal.* The child's tendency to approach or withdraw from new situations such as a new person, a new place, or a new toy.

d.   *Adaptability.* The ease at which the child adapts to new situations.

e.   *Intensity of reaction.* The intensity (strength) of the child's reactions to internal states (such as hunger) and to things in the environment.

f.   *Threshold of responsiveness.* How strong a stimulus has to be to cause the child to respond.

g.   *Quality of mood.* The degree of pleasantness of the child's typical mood.

h.   *Distractibility.* The ease or difficulty with which the child is interrupted while engaged in an activity.

i.   *Attention span.* The amount of time the child remains engaged in an activity.

4.   A baby's temperament influences his/her relationship with parents and caregivers.

C.   Over the first few months of life, developmental changes take place that ready the infant for true social interactions involving mutual give-and-take.

1.   At first the mother or caregiver must orchestrate social exchanges with the infant by

a.   engaging the infant in the interaction;

b.   changing the amount of stimulation in response to the infant's cues; and

c.   being sensitive to the infant's desire to end an interaction.

2.   After about 2 months of age, babies are able to participate in longer social exchanges.

3.   By age 3 to 4 months, infants

  a.   can smile, coo, gurgle, and make other sounds; and
  b.   have good control over their head movements, giving them the ability to turn to interesting stimulation and turn away from stimulation that becomes uninteresting or is too arousing.

4.   By age 4 to 5 months, infants can recognize a parent's/guardian's or regular caregiver's face from among other people and will react specifically to that face.

D.   In the second 6 months of life, marked developments take place.

1.   Babies naturally become more and more interested in exploring their environment and attempting to solve problems.

  a.   Parents/guardians and caregivers influence the infant's exploration of the environment.
  b.   Infants who show more interest and pleasure in exploring the environment and solving problems have parents/guardians or caregivers who are responsive, available, and promote, rather than control, the infant's exploration.

2.   Development of complex emotions.

  a.   After 6 months of age, infants increasingly act to achieve a goal. They can experience

    (1)   the joy of mastering a problem, and
    (2)   the anger of a blocked goal (not being able to have something or do something they desire).

  b.   Infants begin to anticipate others' behavior, and they show the excitement of anticipation. For example, a mother holding a favorite toy indicates to the baby that play is about to begin, and the baby wiggles with excitement.
  c.   The ability to anticipate allows the baby to experience surprise when the unexpected happens.
  d.   Between 7 and 10 months, *stranger distress* typically appears, lasting about 2 to 3 months.

        (1)   The degree of distress varies greatly from infant to infant.

        (2)   The more rapidly and intrusively the stranger approaches, the more likely the baby is to become distressed.

        (3)   Familiar surroundings, presence of the mother, and even a favorite toy can reduce stranger distress.

    e.   Babies in the second 6 months show separation anxiety when parents/guardians leave them and greet parents/guardians joyfully upon their return. These emotions show that the parent/guardian is linked with special, positive feelings.

E.   *Attachment*[1] is an enduring emotional bond between infant and mother developing out of countless hours of interaction.

    1.   Development of attachment

        a.   This emotional bond develops over the first year and continues to develop during toddlerhood and beyond.

        b.   By age 12 months, babies want to be picked up by the mother *specifically,* will seek her out when they are distressed, and appear happier exploring new surroundings when she is present.

        c.   Attachment is different from bonding, the latter of which refers to the mother's tie to the infant in the first days of life.

        d.   Babies will develop an attachment to the person who is consistently available to them.

        e.   Babies can become attached to more than one person.

    2.   Quality of attachment

        a.   Securely attached infants

            (1)   are able to use the mother or primary caregiver as a secure base from which to explore the world;

---

[1] Most research on attachment focuses on the mother and infant. Infants, however, form important attachments to other people, too, including fathers and other caregivers.

           (2)   quickly seek out the mother or primary caregiver when they are upset; and

           (3)   are comforted easily.

  b.   Insecurely attached infants

           (1)   actively avoid interaction with the mother or combine approach and avoidance of the mother in stressful situations;

           (2)   may have parents or caregivers who are

                (a)   inconsistent in providing care;

                (b)   rejecting, indifferent, or emotionally unavailable;

                (c)   frightening or abusive.

3.   Debate continues about the effects of infant child care on attachment.

  a.   By itself, child care of infants probably does not cause insecure attachment.

  b.   The risk of attachment problems may increase when a baby receives full-time child care beginning in the first year, *coupled with* problems at home.

4.   Secure attachment in infancy, compared to insecure attachment, predicts the following:

  a.   A preschooler who is likely to

           (1)   be more self-directed in activities,

           (2)   be more interested in exploring the environment,

           (3)   have better self-control,

           (4)   be more emotionally independent, and

           (5)   show empathy.

  b.   Good preschooler peer relationships including

           (1)   showing positive feelings when engaging and responding to peers,

           (2)   not victimizing others or permitting oneself to be victimized, and

           (3)   showing less aggression.

II.   Toddlers' social-emotional development

A.   The toddler period is a time of transition from infancy to childhood during which dramatic social and emotional changes take place along with major cognitive changes, including the emergence of language and symbolic thought (the ability to think about things that are not present).

B.   Two major tasks of the toddler period are:

1.   To move from near total dependence on parents/guardians and caregivers toward greater independence and self-reliance.

2.   To begin to comply with social rules and values.

C.   Toddlers require less physical closeness to and contact with the caregiver, freeing them to explore the environment more actively.

D.   Toddlers point at and show things to people (especially parents/guardians and familiar caregivers). This enables the toddler to share emotions such as pleasure.

E.   Toddlers use the parent's/guardian's emotional signals (facial expression or tone of voice) as a cue for how to deal with a new situation.

F.   Despite the toddler's push for independence, an overwhelming sense of dependence on the mother or primary caregiver remains.

1.   At the same time the toddler is realizing the choices he/she can make, anxiety about being left by the mother or caregiver peaks.

2.   Separation anxiety is common during the toddler stage. Even brief absences, such as a mother or caregiver leaving the room, can cause distress.

a.   Having a consistent caregiver helps reduce problems in separating from the mother.
b.   Separation is difficult for the mother, too.

G.   Toddlers want to do things with other toddlers.

1.   Play between toddlers revolves around objects, usually giving and taking objects.

2. By playing alongside their peers, toddlers begin to learn skills they need for more complex play in the preschool years.

H. Toddlers are developing a sense of self.

1. They become aware that their own behaviors and intentions are distinct from those of others.

2. They explore the world more actively.

3. They want to do things without help.

I. Toddlers present new demands and challenges for parents/guardians and caregivers.

1. The parent/guardian or caregiver should support the child's movement toward independence while remaining available to step in when the child's capacities are exceeded or safety is threatened.

2. Parents/guardians and caregivers begin to set and maintain rules and limits.

   a. Limits help toddlers feel safe in acting on their newfound independence. A child feels freer to explore if he/she knows the parent will step in if the child needs protection.
   b. Because toddlers often don't know what behavior is acceptable, they frequently test to see which activities are responded to positively or negatively.

3. Toddlers are not distracted as easily from their own goals or plans, which may conflict with those of the parent/guardian or caregiver.

4. Some negativism is a natural outcome of the toddler's increasing independence and self-reliance.

   a. Toddlers frequently say "no."
   b. Children naturally want to comply with their parents' or caregiver's requests and expectations; however, the toddler's desire to cooperate may conflict with the desire to be independent.

III. Preschoolers' social-emotional development

A.   Relationships with peers grow in importance.

1.   The child begins to spend more time with other children and is especially interested in children the same age.

2.   Peer interactions become more complex.   Older preschoolers can

   a.   share a fantasy (as in pretend play),
   b.   make elaborate rules for a game,
   c.   respond to each other's questions, and
   d.   make up and teach new things to do.

3.   Relationships with peers teach children

   a.   how to approach another child and how to start an interaction and keep it going.
   b.   the concepts of fairness, reciprocity (shared obligation), and cooperation.
   c.   to manage aggression.

4.   Peers begin to provide a comparison with the child's own behavior, beliefs, and feelings, which in turn influences the child's self-concept.

B.   Preschoolers begin to achieve skills to regulate their behavior, called *self-regulation*.

1.   Preschoolers can inhibit actions, delay gratification (postpone rewarding themselves), and cope with frustration much more than toddlers can.

2.   When deciding how to act, older preschoolers are able to weigh future consequences.

3.   Preschoolers know how much self-control is needed in different situations and can adjust accordingly.   For example, a child can sit quietly and listen to a story upon request but also can run and shout during outdoor play.

C.   True aggression develops and is common during the preschool years.

    1.   Unlike the hitting, biting, and kicking of toddlers, preschoolers understand the consequences of their actions.

    2.   Most preschool aggression centers on possessing objects.

    3.   During the late preschool and early elementary school years, children behave less aggressively as they learn other ways of handling disputes over objects.

D.   Positive social behaviors become apparent as the preschooler's ability to take the role of others and respond to others' needs grows.

    1.   *Empathy* is the ability to experience the thoughts and feelings of another person. Empathy is fostered in children by nurturing parents or caregivers who

        a.   provide models of empathy and helping toward others;
        b.   clearly explain the consequences for the victim instead of simply scolding the child for hurting others; and
        c.   have expectations for the child regarding kindness.

    2.   *Altruism* is acting unselfishly to help someone else.

E.   Preschoolers strive to be like their parents/guardians or other adults who are important to them. Children adopt the values, beliefs, and thoughts they see in their parents, especially the parent of the same sex.

F.   Preschoolers acquire a sense of being male or female.

    1.   The child identifies with the same-sex parent and other same-sex adults and learns gender-related behaviors, attitudes, and values.

    2.   Sex-typed behavior (behavior more typical of one sex than the other) increases greatly in preschoolers. For example, preschoolers may not want to play with toys they see as appropriate only to the opposite sex.

3.   Preschoolers know they are boys or girls and may prefer to interact with others of the same sex.

4.   By the end of the preschool years, the child understands that gender remains permanent despite changes in age, dress, hair, or behavior. Children learn this about themselves before they apply the idea to others.

G.   Preschoolers' play differs noticeably from toddlers' play in the fantasy it involves. Fantasy play allows children to work through conflicts safely, to master what is frightening or painful, and to try out social roles (playing mommy, daddy, doctor, police officer, teacher, and so on).

H.   Sense of self

1.   By age 3 years or so, children see who they are and expect to stay the same person despite changes in their behavior or in how others respond to them.

2.   Self-esteem (feelings about self) is based on the child's individual experiences. Parents/guardians and care-givers who communicate warmth, empathy, and positive feelings for a child promote self-esteem.

3.   As the preschooler's sense of self continues to develop:

a.   Children adopt the rules and expectations of parents/guardians and caregivers as their own.
b.   Children feel guilty when they do something they know they should not do.

IV.   Implications for child care setting

A.   General social-emotional needs of young children

1.   Be aware of the child's level of social-emotional development.

2.   Recognize that children with disabilities or delays may display uneven development across areas.

3.   Support the child's movement through the various stages of social-emotional development, and be aware that children with disabilities may require extra support.

4. Be continually aware that all children need safe, consistent, and sensitive care.

5. Provide an environment that nurtures and fosters social-emotional development.

     a. Communicate warmth, caring, and empathy to the child.

     b. Emphasize and encourage positive social behaviors.

         (1) Set a good example by modeling kindness, helping, consideration, caring, and cooperation.

         (2) Emphasize and value children helping others.

     c. Plan activities that promote social-emotional development.

B. Important points for infants

1. Respond consistently to a baby's cry by meeting his/her needs.

2. Realize that infants, especially, benefit from care provided by the same familiar person.

3. Respond consistently to infants' needs.

4. Allow yourself enough time to give infants unhurried care.

5. Be aware of young infants' interest in the human face, and provide opportunities for face-to-face interaction during caregiving (feeding, changing, holding, and so on).

6. Promote infants' exploration of the environment.

7. Provide activities and materials that will allow opportunities to master new skills.

C. Important points for toddlers

1. Recognize the value of a consistent caregiver who is responsive to the child's needs, and the same caregiver over time.

2. Minimize the number of different caregivers.

3. Provide an environment that is safe, predictable, helpful, and accepting.

4. Support the toddler's movement toward independence.

    a. Understand that the toddler's quest for independence is natural and necessary.
    b. Step in when toddlers exceed their capabilities or jeopardize their safety.
    c. Be aware of cultural differences in the extent of independence a toddler shows.

5. Set and consistently maintain clear rules and limits.

6. As toddlers require less physical contact with adults, increase nonphysical contact — exchanges of words, smiles, looks.

7. Provide activities to promote learning but do not frustrate the toddler too much.

8. Intervene when necessary to help toddlers calm themselves.

D. Important points for preschoolers

1. Be a consistent and responsive caregiver.

2. Provide opportunities for and encourage relationships with peers.

3. Model empathy and helping.

4. Help children recognize and understand their own and others' feelings.

    a. Help children put their feelings into words.
    b. Talk about anger and appropriate ways to express it.
    c. Help children recognize and respond to the feelings of others.

5. Help children learn to regulate their own emotions and behaviors.

    a. Allow and encourage children to calm themselves.

      b.   Select activities that allow children to express their emotions in a variety of appropriate ways.

      c.   Teach social problem solving by helping children think through and plan their response when they are having a problem with a peer.

      d.   Respond to and provide alternatives to aggression. Don't ignore aggression, but help children think of things they could do instead (use words instead of hitting, and so on).

BIBLIOGRAPHY

Ainsworth, M., Blehar, M., Waters, E., & Wall, S. (1978). *Patterns of attachment*. Hillsdale, NJ: Lawrence Erlbaum.

Bowlby, J. (1969). *Attachment and loss: Vol. 1. Attachment*. New York: Basic Books.

Brazelton, T. B. (1994). *Touchpoints: Your child's emotional and behavioral development*. Reading, MA: Addison-Wesley.

Brazelton, T. B. (1983). *Infants and mothers: Differences in development* (rev.) New York: Delta Books.

Heatherington, E. M., & Parke, R. D. (1986). *Child psychology: A contemporary viewpoint* (3d ed.). New York: McGraw-Hill.

Hyson, M. C. (1994). *The emotional development of young children*. New York: Teachers College Press.

Kuebli, J. (1994). Young children's understanding of everyday emotions. *Young Children, 49*(3), 36-47.

Shure, M. B. (1992). *I can problem-solve: An interpersonal cognitive problem-solving program*. Champaign, IL: Research Press.

Wittmer, D. S., & Honig, A. S. (1994). Encouraging positive social development in young children. *Young Children, 49*(5), 4-12.

Zero to Three. (1992). *Heart Start: The emotional foundations of school readiness*. Arlington, VA: Zero to Three, National Center for Clinical Infant Programs.

SPEECH AND LANGUAGE DEVELOPMENT

I. **Definitions**

    A.   *Communication*: the transmission of a message from one person to another.

    B.   *Language*: the organized system of symbols that people use to communicate with one another.

    C.   *Speech*: the production of the sounds of a language when they are organized into words and word groups.

II. **General principles**

    A.   Young children communicate before they can talk.

        1.   Infants and young children want to communicate.

        2.   Ways to communicate include eye contact, crying, vocalizing, facial expressions, gestures, body postures, speech, and sign language.

    B.   Interaction between adult and child is important for the child's development of speech and language. Children naturally try to communicate with adults. If they do not receive a response, they stop trying to communicate.

    C.   The language learning environment is important.

        1.   Young children communicate about the "here and now."

        2.   An environment offering many experiences and opportunities to explore objects, people, places, and activities supports development of communication skills.

    D.   Language follows general stages and sequences.

        1.   The child's ability to understand language and his/her ability to communicate may develop at different rates.

        2.   Different children move through the stages of language development at different rates.

        3.   In general, children with disabilities move through the same stages and sequences as their communicative skills develop.

4.   Children who use augmentative forms of communication (such as sign language, communication boards or devices) usually move through the same stages as other children.

E.   Difficulties with speech, language, and communication are often seen in young children with disabilities or other special needs.

III. Overview of speech and language development

A.   Infants

1.   First sounds and words include

a.   reflexive sounds and crying,
b.   cooing,
c.   crying that means different things by about 6 months of age,
d.   babbling and playing with sounds,
e.   first words by about 12 months of age,
f.   a vocabulary of about 50 words and starting to put words together, and
g.   using holophrases (for example, *me* for *I want to do it*) and expressions always used as one unit (for example, *timetogo*).

2.   Early uses of sounds, gestures, and words include

a.   eye contact; "anticipating" nipple, bottle, or game; reaching;
b.   other gestures such as pointing, giving, showing;
c.   using sounds and gestures purposefully (by about 12 months of age);
d.   communicative intentions including

(1)   seeking attention,
(2)   requesting objects and actions,
(3)   protesting,
(4)   commenting on objects and actions,
(5)   greeting,
(6)   answering, and
(7)   requesting information;

e.   taking turns with adults, using sounds, gestures, and words.

3. Early understanding is manifested by

    a. responding to familiar people and routines,

    b. responding to name and some familiar words,

    c. using the speaker's intonation and contextual cues to understand,

    d. looking at or giving familiar objects when named (such as patting pictures in a picture book),

    e. following simple directions, and

    f. appearing to understand more than the child is able to say.

B. Toddlers

1. More words and phrases are specifically demonstrated by

    a. using words to replace gestures more often;

    b. expanding vocabulary;

    c. asking simple questions;

    d. using words and phrases to express more meanings such as

        (1) recurrence ("more juice"),

        (2) possession ("mine"),

        (3) location ("up", "there doggie"),

        (4) agent-action ("baby drink"), and

        (5) nonexistence ("all gone ball");

    e. speech becoming clearer but omitting or simplifying some sounds.

2. Words and phrases are used for a variety of purposes including

    a. using words to express communicative intentions that the toddler expressed previously through gestures,

    b. maintaining conversations for more turns,

    c. changing the topic of conversation frequently,

    d. communication revolving around the child, the child's needs and interests,

    e. leading the adult to what the child wants, and

    f. becoming frustrated when not understood.

3. Increase in comprehension skills including

    a. understanding more types of questions,

b. understanding more directions, and
c. still using the speaker's intonation and contextual cues to understand.

C. Preschoolers

1. Expressive language shown by

    a. continuing to expand vocabulary and talk more frequently,
    b. using more complex sentences and using grammatical forms (such as plurals, past tense),
    c. asking many questions,
    d. talking about feelings,
    e. talking about things and events outside of the immediate environment,
    f. being mostly intelligible and fluent by school age but continuing some articulation errors with the letters *l* and *r*.

2. Language development including

    a. using words, phrases, and sentences for a wide variety of purposes,
    b. increasing skills in maintaining conversations by

        (1) acknowledging partner's turn,
        (2) using repetition to maintain a topic,
        (3) modifying language when talking to a younger child,
        (4) being more aware of partner's level of understanding;

    c. applying basic grammatical rules to everything, sometimes incorrectly (for example, having learned the basic use of the "- ed" form for past tense, the child may say "seed" instead of "saw," "doed" instead of "did").

3. Comprehension as manifested by

    a. understanding more words, including verbs and adjectives,
    b. understanding prepositions,
    c. following directions that have several steps,
    d. beginning to understand time, space, and speed.

IV. **Supporting the development of communication skills**

    A.   General guidelines

        1.   Young children need conversational partners who are responsive, consistent, and predictable.

        2.   Children use strategies to learn language.

            a.   Children use what they already know and the contextual information (what the adult is pointing at, what usually happens next, and so on) to help them figure out what is being said.

            b.   Children pay attention to what is interesting or new about objects, people, and events.

            c.   Children learn that if they vocalize (talk), people will pay attention to them.

            d.   Some children use imitation to learn language.

            e.   Some children use an analytic or trial-and-error method to learn language.

            f.   Children may use all or some of these strategies.

    B.   Considerations for infants

        1.   Assume a face-to-face position with the infant.

        2.   Use repetitive play routines and rituals to help infants learn to communicate and take turns ("so big," "patty cake").

        3.   Respond to and interpret the infant's signals as meaningful (for example, infant cries after waking up, and you say, "Oh, you want to get up").

        4.   Have "conversations" with the infant; pause for the infant's turn (pick up the infant and say, "Here we go"; the infant smiles, and you say, "Now you're up," the infant gurgles, and you say "That's a happy baby").

        5.   Imitate the infant's sounds, gestures, or actions as a way of taking turns at the child's developmental level.

6. Introduce books; let the infant explore the book; name the pictures (read the book with the infant) for a short time.

7. Label the infant's experiences, and describe the infant's actions using single words or short sentences.

8. Use toys and objects that do things and that the infant can play with.

C. Considerations for toddlers

1. Imitate what the child says and then say a little bit more (the child says "big dog," and you say "a big, brown dog").

2. Provide interesting toys, objects, and activities to talk about.

3. Say new words and pair them with the object, action, or event.

4. Describe what you are doing, thinking, or feeling; this self-talk gives the child new information.

5. Use familiar play routines, games, and songs to teach new words and concepts (for example, insert some new words into a familiar song).

6. Explore parks, zoos, grocery stores, with young children; talk about what you see and do both during and after the field trip.

7. Create opportunities for the child to make requests and initiate conversations (for example, if a child can see a toy but not reach it, the child may ask for it).

8. Repeat information in slightly different ways (for example, say, "it's time to paint," "we need our paint brushes to paint," "okay, let's paint").

D. Considerations for preschoolers

1. Use the child's own play as language learning opportunities; observe, participate, and converse.

2. Comment and expand on what the child has to say.

3. Model language skills.

4. Continue to explore the world through field trips.

5. Include new experiences such as cooking and simple science experiments.

6. Plan for new vocabulary or concepts to accompany themes or activities.

7. Continue to read books; help the child "read"; retell the story; or create stories.

8. Provide opportunities and materials for symbolic or dramatic play.

9. Even when young children are on the go, help them learn language; mini-conversations can be language learning opportunities if they are matched to the child's interests.

V.   Implications for children with disabilities and special needs

A. A child may have speech or language disabilities alone or in association with other disabilities.

B. Speech and language disabilities can range from mild to severe.

C. The caregiver should be aware of the dialect and language used in the child's home so cultural differences are not mistaken for problems in language development.

D. Early identification of speech and language difficulties is critical.

E. Some children may need to use augmentative forms of communication (such as sign language, communication boards or devices). Caregivers should be familiar with the devices and how they are used.

F. The caregiver should consult the child's specialists and other team members to plan speech and language learning activities.

BIBLIOGRAPHY

Buchoff, R. (1994). Joyful voices: Facilitating language growth through rhythmic response to chants. *Young Children, 49*(4), 26-30.

Jones, H. A., & Warren, S. F. (1991). Enhancing engagement in early language teaching. *Teaching Exceptional Children, 23*(4), 48-50.

Mulligan, S. A., Green, K. M., Morris, S. L., Maloney, T. J., McMurray, D., & Kittelson-Aldred, T. (1992). *Integrated child care.* Tucson, AZ: Communication Skill Builders.

Ostrosky, M. M., & Kaiser, A. P. (1991). Preschool classroom environments that promote communication. *Teaching Exceptional Children, 23*(4), 6-10.

Parette, H. P., Dunn, N. S., & Reichert Hoge, D. (1995). Low-cost communication devices for children with disabilities and their family members. *Young Children, 50*(6), 75-81.

RESOURCES

American Speech-Language-Hearing Association, 10801 Rockville Pike, Rockville, MD 20852; (301) 897-5700 (Voice/TDD)

National Center for Stuttering, 200 E. 33rd St., New York, NY 10016; 1-800-221-2488 or (212) 537-1460

II. CHRONIC CONDITIONS

Auditory Impairment

Cerebral Palsy (CP)

Spina Bifida

Visual Impairment

Adapting Learning Activities for Children with Physical/Sensory Impairments

Down Syndrome

Mental Retardation

Fetal Alcohol Syndrome

Adapting Learning for Children with Cognitive Delays

Prenatal Exposure to Drugs

Pediatric HIV Infection

Emotional Problems

Congenital Heart Defects

Major Respiratory Diseases in Children

Apnea Monitoring

Children with Seizures

AUDITORY IMPAIRMENT

I. Defining and detecting auditory impairment

A. Auditory impairment is an inability to hear sounds and speech adequately, which in young children hinders learning to understand and produce speech.

   1. The hearing loss may be in one or both ears or may be worse in one ear than the other ear.

   2. Hearing losses may be stable, progressive (slowly but continually getting worse), or fluctuating.

B. Extent of hearing loss

   1. The amount or degree of hearing loss and its effect on a child vary from mild to profound.

      a. Most people with a hearing deficit have some remaining hearing.
      b. Mild hearing loss is difficult to identify because of its subtle effect on the child.

   2. A child with profound hearing loss does not respond to any amount of sound; without intervention, language and speech will not develop normally.

C. Incidence

   1. About 22,000 infants are born with or acquire permanent hearing loss each year.[1]

   2. About 1% of all children have a persistent hearing loss (not caused temporarily by infection or other impediment).

   3. Profound hearing loss or total deafness affects about 2 in 1,000 children.[2]

---

[1] Source: *Hearing in Children* (4th ed.), by J. L. Northern & M. P. Downs (Baltimore: Williams & Wilkins, 1991).

[2] Source: *Children with Disabilities: A Medical Primer* (3d ed.), by M. L. Batshaw & Y. M. Perret (Baltimore: Paul H. Brookes, 1992).

D. Detection

    1. Deafness may run in families, so, if that is the case, infants should be checked as early as possible.

    2. Because hearing loss seldom has any visible signs and associated behaviors can be misleading, children with undiagnosed hearing loss often are mislabeled as inattentive, uncooperative, disinterested, or as having mental retardation.

    3. Hearing loss should be identified as early as possible to permit early intervention.

    4. Because of the potentially devastating effects of hearing loss and the benefits of early identification and treatment, *all* children should receive a hearing screening at least once a year.

II. Types of hearing loss

A. Conductive hearing loss

    1. In this type of impairment, sound is blocked or is not transmitted to the inner ear.

    2. It has two main causes:

        a. Ear wax (cerumen) or foreign objects fill and block outer ear canal, leaving no passageway for sound.
        b. Ear infection (otitis media) stiffens the ear drum so it does not transfer sounds inward.

    3. Hearing losses range from mild to moderate impairment and possibly vary from day to day.

    4. This is the type of loss that reduces the loudness, but not necessarily the clarity, of sounds.

    5. It usually can be improved with medical or surgical treatment.

B. Sensorineural hearing loss

    1. In this type of impairment, the brain does not understand sound that reaches the inner ear. In some cases the signals reaching the brain are loud enough but are unclear or distorted.

2.   Hearing losses range from mild to profound.

3.   The loss is usually permanent (cannot be improved medically or surgically).

4.   Hearing aids are recommended.

C.   Mixed hearing loss: a combination of conductive and sensorineural hearing loss

III.   Effect of hearing loss on development

A.   Congenital (inborn) or early-onset hearing loss will limit the development of a language base, or symbol system, in the brain, needed for thinking and processing information.   A sign system of some nature *must* be introduced as early as possible for maximum cognitive development and to decrease the chance of behavior problems developing.

B.   Piaget's stages of thinking development:[3]

1.   Stage 1 — Sensorimotor (0-18 months):   Child learns about objects and events in environment.

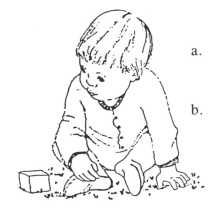

a.   The child with hearing impairment learns that objects can be seen, touched, and smelled, but perhaps not heard.

b.   Development of cause, time, and space is visual.

---

[3] Adapted from S. Watkins, *Developing Cognition in Young Hearing-Impaired Children*, by permission of SKI HI Institute, Logan, UT.

2.   Stage 2 — Preoperational (2-7 years): Child learns language.

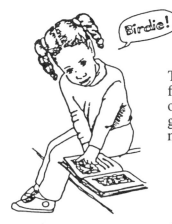

The child with a hearing impairment forms a mental picture of an object but often attaches a visual symbol (pointing, gesturing) instead of a spoken word to the mental picture.

C.   Children with hearing loss are not able to understand the speech of others.

D.   Speech is delayed or not understandable.

E.   Social and emotional skills may become a problem as the child recognizes his/her difficulties in communication.

F.   Prelinguistic hearing impairment or deafness (present before language develops)

1.   A sign system should be introduced when the child is about 6 months of age, as infants will begin to make signs at that age.

2.   Deaf children of parents who are deaf make greater progress if parents teach signing early.

3.   American Sign Language (ASL or Ameslan) has most of the features of spoken English.

4.   An oral system versus a sign approach is controversial. Some therapists use both in what is known as *total communication*.

IV.   Applicable legislation

A.   The Americans with Disabilities Act (ADA) requires places of "public accommodation," including centers and preschools, to ensure or provide for effective and accurate communication unless an undue burden or fundamental alteration would result. This is subject to interpretation, but the preschool or center may be responsible for arranging and paying for a sign language interpreter, given reasonable advance notice.

B. ADA requires telephone companies to establish a relay service to translate from speech to teletypewriter for individuals with hearing loss.

C. The Individuals with Disabilities Education Act (IDEA) requires that each participating state must organize an Interagency Coordinating Council and select a lead agency responsible for ensuring the identification and service planning of children ages birth to 21 who have or are at risk for developmental disabilities. This includes children with auditory impairment.

V. Screening and diagnosis

A. Early identification/screening

1. A child should have a formal hearing evaluation if he/she has any of the high-risk factors for hearing loss listed in the History form at the end of this module.

2. Any indicators of possible hearing loss should be recorded. (see History form at end of unit).

3. The parent/guardian should be referred to Child Find, County Public Health Office, or local audiologist for information on and availability of hearing screening/diagnosis.

B. Professionals involved in diagnosis

1. Audiologists: have a master's degree or doctorate in the study of hearing.

2. Ear, nose, and throat (ENT) physicians: doctors with additional specialized training in the evaluation and medical and surgical treatment of the ears, nose, and throat.

3. Speech/language pathologists: have a master's degree or doctorate in the study of evaluation and therapy techniques for speech and language development.

C.   Diagnosis

1.   For infants, toddlers, and young children, sound can be played through the ear and measured by reception in the auditory area of the brain. If low or no response is detected, a hearing deficit may be present.

2.   *Audiometry* measures the softest individual tones and speech sounds a child can hear and the clarity of what he/she hears.

3.   *Tympanometry* tests the ear drum and middle ear system to determine proper sound transfer to the inner ear. This is done by bouncing sound off the ear drum and measuring the amount of sound reflected back to the machine.

4.   Medical evaluation is done to determine the cause of the hearing loss and any treatment that may improve the child's hearing or keep the loss from worsening.

5.   Speech/language evaluation is conducted to determine what effect the hearing loss may have had on speech/language development and determine the need for therapy.

VI.   (Re)Habilitation

A.   *Habilitation* is the teaching of new skills to help the child reach age-appropriate developmental milestones.

B.   *Rehabilitation* works toward restoration of lost functioning.

C.   Hearing aids

1.   Caregivers should receive training in the operation of the type(s) of hearing aid present in the center.

2.   Parents/guardians are to leave a pack of batteries at the center.

3.   Special helmets or bonnets are available to keep hearing aids in the child's ears.

D.   FM systems

1.   Caregivers should be trained in the operation of any FM systems used.

2. Options include: direct input, loop, silhouette, external receiver/headphones.

E. Auditory training

   1. is therapy to strengthen listening skills,

   2. makes best use of remaining hearing,

   3. follows normal developmental patterns.

F. Speech therapy: specialized, intense training to develop normal speech and language skills

VII. Special care needs

A. Background noise

   1. Turn the radio and TV down or off when talking with the child.

   2. Do not talk with the child when the faucet is running or the vacuum cleaner is being used.

   3. Take some time in a quiet place when you can read to or talk with the child.

B. Attention

   1. Before speaking, gain the child's attention.

   2. Check frequently that you still have the child's attention.

   3. Maintain good eye contact.

   4. Be sure the child can see your face and hands easily when you are speaking or reading aloud.

C. Talking skills

   1. Talk a lot (children with hearing loss need more input), but do not dominate the conversation. Allow the child to respond or initiate communication, too.

   2. Speak clearly, a little more slowly, and a little louder than usual, but try to keep your tone natural.

3. If the child does not understand, repeat your statement, perhaps using different words.

4. Speak at the child's level of functioning. Don't use big words or long phrases that may be confusing to the child.

D. Nonverbal communication

1. Use visual cues and gestures as reinforcers to what you are saying.

2. Use a lot of facial expressions to convey mood or tone.

3. Try to communicate as much as possible at the child's eye level.

4. If a child with profound hearing loss uses sign language, learn a few basic signs.

E. Ear infections (otitis media)

1. Maintain good, frequent communication with parent/ guardian.

a. Ask parent/guardian to let you know when the child has an ear infection, and any medication prescribed.[4]

b. Encourage parent/guardian to talk with you about signs and symptoms of ear infections to watch for in the child, such as

(1) upper respiratory infection
(2) teething
(3) tugging at ear or rubbing side of the face
(4) drainage from the ear
(5) complaints of pain in or around the ear

---

[4] Administration of medication is generally regarded as an invasive procedure and, as such, is a nursing task that may be subject to statutory provisions or to regulations established by your State's Nursing Board. If this is the case, legislation or regulatory guidelines may be in place that determine whether or not and how this task may be delegated to a non-health-licensed individual (other than the child's parent or guardian). For the safety of the children, and due to the risk of personal and agency liability, you are urged to contact your State Board of Nursing to inquire about the status of delegation of invasive procedures in your state.

2. Ensure that medications are given on time and completely even if the symptoms have gone away.

3. Preventing ear infections:

    a. Keep the child dry, fed nutritionally, and allow adequate sleep.
    b. Keep the child away from others with ear infections and upper respiratory infections (URI) as much as possible.
    c. Keep the child away from smoke and other respiratory irritants.
    d. Do not put infants down to sleep with a bottle.

BIBLIOGRAPHY

Batshaw, M. L., & Perret, Y. M. (1992). *Children with disabilities.* Baltimore: Paul H. Brookes.

Bess, F., & Hall, J. (1992). *Screening children for auditory function.* Nashville, TN: Bill Wilkerson Center Press.

Northern, J., & Downs, M. (1991). *Hearing in children* (4th ed.). Baltimore: Williams and Wilkens.

RESOURCES

Alexander Graham Bell Association for the Deaf, 3417 Volta Place NW, Washington, DC 20007; (202) 337-5220 (Voice/TDD)

American Academy of Audiology, 1735 North Lynn, Suite 950, Arlington, VA 22209; 1-800-222-2336

American Association of the Deaf and Blind, 814 Thayer Avenue, Silver Spring, MD 20910; (301) 555-1212 or (301) 588-6545 (TDD)

American Speech, Language, Hearing Association, 10801 Rockville Pike, Rockville, MD 20852; (301) 897-5700

Hearing Aid Helpline, 20361 Middlebelt Road, Livonia, MI 48152; 1-800-521-5247

National Information Center on Deafness, Gallaudet University, 800 Florida Avenue NE, Washington, DC 20002-3695; (202) 651-5051 or (202) 651-5052 (TDD)

HISTORY FOR IDENTIFICATION OF
HEARING AND MIDDLE EAR DYSFUNCTION

Child's Name_____ Age_____ Date_____

High-Risk Factors:

Yes ____ No ____   Family history of congenital or early
                         sensorineural hearing loss

Yes ____ No ____   Congenital infection known or suspected to
                         be associated with sensorineural hearing loss
                         such as toxoplasmosis, syphilis, rubella,
                         cytomegalovirus, and herpes

Yes ____ No ____   Craniofacial anomalies

Yes ____ No ____   Birth weight less than 1500 grams (3.3
                         pounds)

Yes ____ No ____   Hyperbilirubinemia at a level exceeding
                         indication for exchange transfusion

Yes ____ No ____   Ototoxic medications used for more than 5
                         days

Yes ____ No ____   Bacterial meningitis

Yes ____ No ____   Severe depression at birth (Apgar scores of
                         0-3 at 5 minutes)

Yes ____ No ____   Prolonged mechanical ventilation (more than
                         10 days)

Yes ____ No ____   Other findings associated with a syndrome
                         known to include sensorineural hearing loss

Other Information:

Yes ____ No ____   Recent or current ear pain

Yes ____ No ____   Recent or current ear discharge/drainage

Yes ____ No ____   Auditory developmental delay

Yes ____ No ____   Speech/language developmental delay

Visual Inspection: Note any malformation or abnormality of the
                         head and neck that has not received previous
                         medical evaluation

Source: Colorado Academy of Audiology, (303) 351-1595

CEREBRAL PALSY (CP)

I.   Definition/description

A.   Cerebral palsy (CP) is a general term referring to a variety of conditions.

B.   All cases have in common an impairment in muscle coordination, resulting in an inability to maintain normal posture and balance and to perform normal movement and skills.

C.   Muscle tone may be

     1.   *hypertonic* (high muscle tone; rigid); or

     2.   *hypotonic* (low muscle tone; floppy); or

     3.   some combination of both.

D.   Cerebral palsy is caused by some injury or damage to the brain before, during, or after birth, including

     1.   genetic/inherited/chromosomal factors,

     2.   trauma to the brain when growing in the uterus,

     3.   infections in the uterus,

     4.   lack of oxygen to the brain at birth,

     5.   intracranial hemorrhage (bleeding within the brain),

     6.   meningitis in childhood, or

     7.   poisoning;

     8.   specific cause unknown (half of the cases).

E.   Cerebral palsy also is associated with prematurity and low birth weight.

II.   General characteristics and prevalance

A.   Characteristically, CP

     1.   is noncontagious (cannot be transmitted to others),

2.   is nonprogressive (but the condition may look worse as the child gets older and larger),

3.   is incurable but not fatal,

4.   can improve with proper treatment (early intervention is most effective), and

5.   often is not identifiable at birth; quality of infant's motor development also may change over the course of infancy.

B.   CP is the most common physical impairment in children (.6 to 2.4 per 1,000 children)[1]

III.   Classifications[2]

A.   Spastic or pyramidal cerebral palsy (most common type of CP), characterized by

1.   hypertonicity of extremities and hypotonicity of neck and trunk,

2.   persistent primitive reflexes,

3.   poor control of posture, balance, and coordinated movement,

4.   joint and bone deformities,

5.   slow, labored movements,

6.   varied amount of movement, and can affect body parts differently, as

a.   *quadriplegia:* all four extremities involved
b.   *diplegia:* legs more involved than arms
c.   *hemiplegia:* one side of body, both arm and leg, more involved

---

[1] *Children with Disabilities* edited by M. Batshaw and Y. M. Perret (Baltimore: Paul H. Brookes Publishing, 1991), p. 443.

[2] Some children have a mixed type of cerebral palsy and show characteristics of more than one type.

B. Dyskinetic or athetoid cerebral palsy, characterized by

    1. slow, wormlike, writhing, involuntary movements; and

    2. absent during sleep; aggravated by stress.

C. Ataxic cerebral palsy characterized by

    1. irregular muscle action and lack of muscle coordination

    2. broad-based, lurching gait; problems with balance

    3. dislike of being moved off mid-line

D. Associated disabilities include (any or all)

    1. sensory impairment(s),

    2. visual problems related to muscle imbalance,

    3. hearing problems,

    4. learning disabilities,

    5. seizures,

    6. mental retardation, and

    7. communication/speech problems.

IV. **Common manifestations of cerebral palsy**

A. Delayed gross-motor and fine-motor development

B. Abnormal motor performance

C. Alterations of muscle tone

D. Abnormal postures

E. Persistence of primitive reflexes

F. If facial muscles are involved, the result may be

    1. low tone with open mouth,

    2. smile that look like a grimace, and/or

    3. interference with eating, drinking, and speaking.

G.   Children with CP often do not cuddle easily.

    1.   They may arch away or may not have the ability to hold on.

    2.   These movement patterns may make you think they do not want to be held.

V.   Special care needs

A.   Special equipment and therapy

    1.   Be familiar with special chairs (including wheelchairs and positioning devices).

    2.   Know the purpose of braces/splints.

    3.   Know how to use any special feeding utensils.

    4.   Adhere to any speech, physical, and occupational therapy techniques individualized according to the child's need.

B.   Caregiver/staff interactions

    1.   Talk about the child's needs.

    2.   List routine procedures for the child.

    3.   Use recommended techniques in positioning, feeding, and general care.

    4.   Determine what positions/activities may cause or increase abnormal movements in the child, and avoid these.

C.   Overall goals

    1.   Establish movement, communication, and self-help skills.

        a.   Use correct positions.
        b.   Work for symmetry.
        c.   Work toward mid-line of body.
        d.   Provide only as much assistance as necessary.

    2.   Work to achieve optimum appearance and integration of motor functioning.

3. Follow procedures to prevent deformities.

4. Strive to have associated defects corrected as early and effectively as possible.

5. Provide educational and social opportunities for the child.

D. How to accomplish goals

1. Provide extra calories to meet the energy demands of increased muscle activity.

2. Encourage sitting, crawling, and walking at appropriate stages according to the therapy plan.

3. Provide incentives for the child to move around.

4. Communication

a. Talk slowly to the child in a conversational way.
b. Give the child plenty of time to respond.
c. Learn the child's unique communication signals.
d. Always tell the child what you are going to do with him/her.
e. Use articles and pictures to reinforce speech.

5. Apply and use braces correctly.

6. Provide a safe environment.

7. Use restraints when the child is in a chair or vehicle.

8. Select age-appropriate toys and activities that allow the child maximum participation.

9. Do not persist too long to accomplish goals; work slowly and avoid rapid movement.

10. Adapt utensils, food, and clothing to facilitate self-help.

11. Be alert to evidence of fatigue.

12. Avoid forcing or pulling on a child's limb to get it into position.

13. Change the child's position regularly.

a. Place the child in positions so he/she can be in contact with the rest of the world.
b. Include the child in the group as a participant, not just an onlooker.
c. Use good body mechanics when picking up and carrying the child.

14. Try not to engage in activities that reinforce the child's dysfunctional motor patterns (for example, baby walkers tend to encourage stiff legs and walking on toes).

15. Provide adaptive equipment as needed.

BIBLIOGRAPHY

Alexander, R., Boehme, R., & Cupps, B. (1993). *Normal development of functional motor skills, the first year of life.* San Antonio, TX: Therapy Skill Builders.

Batshaw, M. L., & Perret, Y. M. (1994). *Children with handicaps: A medical primer* (3d ed.). Baltimore: Paul H. Brookes Publishing.

Kapute, A., & Accardo, P. (1991). *Developmental disabilities in infancy and childhood.* Baltimore: Paul H. Brookes Publishing.

Lynch, E. W., & Hanson, M. J. (Eds.) (1992). *Developing cross-cultural competence: A guide for working with young children and their families.* Baltimore: Paul H. Brookes Publishing.

Miller, S. E., & Schaumberg, K. (1988). Physical education activities for children with cerebral palsy. *Teaching Exceptional Children, 20*(2), 9-11.

Schaeffler, C. (1988). Making toys accessible for children with cerebral palsy. *Teaching Exceptional Children, 20*(3), 26-28.

Schleichkorn, J. (1983). *Coping with cerebral palsy: Questions parents often ask.* Austin, TX: Pro-Ed.

RESOURCES

American Academy for Cerebral Palsy and Developmental Medicine, 1910 Byrd Ave., Suite 118, P. O. Box 11086, Richmond, VA 23230-1086, (804) 282-0036

United Cerebral Palsy Association, 7 Penn Plaza, Suite 804, New York, NY 10001; 1-800-USA-IUCP

SPINA BIFIDA

I. Definitions

A. *Spina bifida:* a birth defect of the spinal column that results in muscle weakness or paralysis or both, as well as a lack of sensation below the area of the defect.

B. *Hydrocephalus:* a condition in which fluid in the brain is not absorbed properly; also known as "water on the brain."[1]

   1. Is present in 80% to 90% of spina bifida cases and also in some children without spina bifida.

   2. A *shunt* or catheter is inserted surgically to drain excess fluid from the brain.

   3. Warning signs of shunt malfunction[2]

      a. Infants

         (1) increased head size
         (2) bulging fontanel ("soft spot")
         (3) swelling along the shunt tract
         (4) less appetite; vomiting
         (5) "sunsetting" (downward gaze of eyes or eyes become crossed)
         (6) irritability
         (7) drowsiness; lower level of arousal/consciousness
         (8) seizure(s)

      b. Toddlers and preschoolers

         (1) headaches
         (2) swelling along shunt tract
         (3) loss of appetite; vomiting
         (4) irritability
         (5) drowsiness, lower level of arousal/consciousness
         (6) decline of developmental milestones

---

[1] Hydrocephalus occurs in some children without spina bifida as well.

[2] The symptoms listed may be present in a child, but not all children will exhibit all the warning signs. For each child, the parents can best tell the usual sequence of signs and symptoms of a shunt malfunction.

       (7)   seizure(s)
       (8)   weakness/paralysis

II.   Incidence and causes

A.   Spina bifida occurs in about 1 of every 1,000 births.[3]

B.   The defect happens during the first month of pregnancy.

C.   The cause is unknown; but several different factors or a combination of factors may be involved.

III. Outcomes

A.   Although spina bifida is a complex disorder, the child's overall health may be good and intelligence can be expected to be normal or close to it.

B.   Children with spina bifida may and do attend general education classes, participate in recreational activities, and go on to become productive members of society as adults.

IV. Orthopedic deformities and care

A.   Orthopedic care starts at birth and continues throughout life, focusing on both *prevention* and *correction* of defects.

B.   Affected areas

    1.   Dislocated hip(s)

       a.   Instability of the hip joint is the result.
       b.   If not corrected, the child's ability to walk may be affected.

    2.   Feet and knee deformities

       a.   A wide variety of deformities may be present because of less control and sensation in the legs and feet.
       b.   If nerves were lost prior to birth, limbs may be smaller because they weren't stimulated to develop.

---

[3] Source: Spina Bifida Association, 1995.

3. Muscle weakness

    a. The extent varies from slight weakness to complete loss of function in the legs.

    b. Weakness also may be present to some extent in the trunk and upper body, depending on the location of the spinal cord defect.

    c. Rolling, sitting up, crawling, and walking may be delayed.

C. Management consists of

1. physical therapy, exercise, and

2. bracing

D. Warning signs of orthopedic injury and pressure sores include

1. swelling of a limb,

2. deformity of a limb (change in the usual appearance of the limb), and/or

3. redness around the area.

V. Other conditions commonly associated with spina bifida

A. Neurogenic bladder

1. Definition: loss of voluntary control of the bladder

2. Description

    a. In children with flaccid (limp) bladder, the muscles do not empty the bladder, and the urine dribbles out constantly.

    b. Urine also may back up into the kidneys and damage them.

    c. Children with spastic (irritable) bladder may have intermittent leakage (may come and go).

3. Management may consist of

    a. *Crede method* of manual expression of urine

    b. *indwelling catheter* (draining tube left in place in the bladder: not recommended for long-term use, and/or

    c. clean intermittent catheterization.

4. Warning signs of urinary tract infection (are

    a. fever,
    b. foul smelling urine,
    c. blood in urine,
    d. nausea, vomiting, loss of appetite, and
    e. irritability.

B. Neurogenic bowel

    1. Definition: weakness or loss of voluntary control of rectal sphincter

    2. Description

        a. Can cause constipation, diarrhea, and bowel accidents.
        b. Children with neurogenic bladder do not necessarily have neurogenic bowel.

    3. Management may consist of

        a. diet modification (high fluid and fiber intake),
        b. medications,
        c. bowel training (regular emptying of the bowels by various means), and/or
        d. colostomy

            (1) may be necessary if the above measures are not successful
            (2) rare in early childhood

VI. Special care needs

A. Skin care

    1. Be aware that, because of lack of pain sensation, the child may not notice an injury to the skin.

    2. Pay close attention to skin condition, and point out any suspicions to parent/guardian.

B. Stimulation

    1. Physical

        a. Increase tactile (touch) stimulation to increase body awareness.

b. Make adaptations so the room, toys, and materials are accessible and safe for a child with limitations in mobility.

2. Cognitive

a. Be aware of short attention span and distractibility in some children with spina bifida.
b. Provide learning environments that encourage their participation.

C. Diet

1. Be aware of nutritional problems posed by limited mobility plus people's tendency to equate food and love, which may lead to child's obesity, making mobility even more difficult.

2. Provide children with spina bifida good nutrition in general, and adequate calcium for bone growth and density.

3. Provide plenty of fluid intake.

D. Social needs

1. To be as normal and competent as possible.

2. To be in the mainstream of family and school life.

3. To be disciplined like other children.

BIBLIOGRAPHY

McLone, D. (1986). *An introduction to spina bifida.* Washington, DC: Spina Bifida Association of America. (booklet)

Smith, K. (1990). Bowel and bladder management of the child with myelomeningocele in the school setting. *Journal of Pediatric Health Care, 4*(4), 175-180.

Williamson, G. (1987). *Children with spina bifida: Early intervention and preschool programming.* Baltimore: Paul H. Brookes.

RESOURCES

March of Dimes Birth Defects Foundation, National Foundation — March of Dimes, 1275 Mamaroneck Ave., White Plains, NY 10605; (914) 428-7100 (including Spanish)

Spina Bifida Association of America, 4590 MacArthur Blvd. NW, Suite 250, Washington, DC 20007-4226; 1-800-621-3141 or (202) 944-3285

VISUAL IMPAIRMENT

I. **Definitions**

A. Visual impairment: loss of eyesight as a result of damage to the eye itself, the optic nerve along its pathway, or visual centers of the brain.

   1. *Congenital:* born with a malformation or visual defect.

   2. *Adventitious:* vision present at birth but lost because of acquired disease, tumor, or trauma.

B. Legal definition of blindness

   1. Visual acuity less than 20/200 in the better eye with best possible correction. (Example: child with proper glasses has to stand 20 feet away to see what child with 20/20 acuity can see from 200 feet away.)

   2. Visual field is restricted to 20° or less from normal 180° visual field in the better eye (like looking through a tube).

C. Total blindness: complete loss of vision

D. Low vision or partially sighted

   1. Some functional vision remains

   2. Some modifications of materials and environment for learning are needed.

   3. Range is from primarily visual learner to relying primarily on hearing, touch, and other senses for learning.

II. **Possible effects of visual impairment**

A. Visual acuity (clarity) is reduced.

   1. Myopia (nearsighted): close objects are seen best.

   2. Hyperopia (farsighted): objects that are far away are seen best; close objects are hard to see.

B. Visual field (total area seen) is reduced because of:

    1. Tunnel vision (like looking through a straw) OR

    2. Blind spots (scotomas) OR

    3. Peripheral vision (sees on only one or both sides; unclear or reduced central viewing).

C. Oculomotor problems (uncoordinated eye muscle movements)

    1. Strabismus ("crossed" eyes or one eye moves out of focus; eyes do not focus on the same object at the same time)

    2. Amblyopia ("lazy eye"; one eye is not being used)

    3. Nystagmus (eyes move in quick, rhythmic jerks)

D. Unreliable visual processing

    1. Cortical visual impairment (brain is not able to receive and interpret visual information)

    2. No structural abnormality in the eyeball

E. Reduced sensitivity to contrast (difficulty discriminating lightness and darkness)

    1. Sensitivity to glare and bright light

    2. Impairment in color vision or discrimination

III. Prevalence

A. About five children in 1,000 have some visual impairment.

B. About 52,000 people in the United States are classified as legally blind.[1]

C. More than three-fourths of children with visual impairment have some useful (functional) vision.

---

[1] Source: American Printing House for the Blind, P.O. Box 6085, Louisville, KY 40206

D.   More than half of children with visual impairment have an additional disability (cerebral palsy, hearing, neurological involvement, cognitive).

E.   Most common visual disorders in 0-5 year ages are:

1.   Cortical visual impairment

2.   Retinopathy of prematurity

3.   Congenital (inborn) malformations

4.   Oculomotor (visual-motor) problems

5.   Cataracts

F.   Various disorders of the retina, thought to be caused by the mother's prenatal substance abuse, are gaining ground. Optic nerve hypoplasia ranks third in one study.

IV.   Signs of visual impairment

A.   Squinting or frowning when looking

B.   Jerky eye movements

C.   Extreme sensitivity to light

D.   Eyes not working or moving together

E.   Excessive eye blinking or eye rubbing

F.   Strange head posturing or head thrusting to see; covering or shutting one eye

G.   Not visually attentive to objects or surroundings or cannot hold visual attention more than a few seconds before looking away

H.   Bumping into obstacles; missing drop-offs or stairs

I.   Holding objects very close to eyes to see

J.   Eyes frequently tearing, red, swollen, or encrusted

K.   Complaints of dizziness, nausea, or headache following close eye work

V.   **Screening and diagnosis**

    A.   General screening or exam for suspected vision problem

       1.   By preschool nurse or special education coordinator

       2.   By family physician, pediatrician, or health services coordinator

       3.   By preschool vision screening request to local chapter of National Society for the Prevention of Blindness or other paraprofessional volunteer group

    B.   Eye specialists

       1.   Ophthalmologist

           a.   Doctor of medicine
           b.   Diagnoses and treats eye disease and can perform surgery
           c.   Can prescribe eyeglasses and medication

       2.   Optometrist

           a.   Can prescribe glasses
           b.   Can do low-vision exams
           c.   In some cases can provide vision training therapy with a vision therapist for problems such as "lazy eye"

    C.   Local service agencies

       1.   Local Child Find office

       2.   State Department of Education, Early Childhood Department, Department of Visual Impairment

       3.   State Social Services (rehabilitation departments in many states have infant and preschool resources for children with visual impairment)

       4.   Specialized programs

           a.   State schools for individuals who are blind and have visual impairment
           b.   Private agencies can provide inservices, direct services, and written resources for Head Starts, preschools

VI. **Impact of vision impairment on development**

    A.   90% of learning comes through vision; therefore, a visual loss affects development in all areas.

    B.   Generally more time is needed to attain developmental skills, but there is wide diversity; all children are different.

    C.   Developmental sequence may be different.

    D.   Fine and gross motor development is area of greatest delay; requires many adaptations and one-to-one learning.

    E.   Cognitive status is difficult to ascertain in early years because so much of early learning is visual; children often are misdiagnosed with mental impairment when they have not had experiences that would allow them to develop concepts.

VII. **Unique learning needs**

    A.   Sensory development to compensate for visual loss

        1.   Auditory

            a.   Sounds are cues to activity or object.
            b.   Sounds provide clues to direction and distance of sounds.

        2.   Functional vision

            a.   Functional vision localizes to light/objects.
            b.   It is secondary to or verifies other sensory information.
            c.   Sometimes called "travel vision."

        3.   Tactile (touch)

            a.   The child substitutes touch for vision loss to determine size, shape, texture, temperature, and weight of materials.
            b.   Tactile sensitivity (sensitivity to touch) is common.

        4.   Olfactory (smell) and gustatory (taste)

            a.   The child uses these senses in real experiences.

         b.   The child uses these senses to identify people, objects, places.

    5.   Sense of body position or movement

         a.   The child develops muscle memory (examples: keeping head up, jumping).
         b.   The child develops spatial concepts (examples: up, through, over).

B.   Unifying experiences

    1.   Understanding parts-to-whole relationship: the child with visual impairment may receive only bits and pieces of sensory information. (Examples: a child's concept of "car" comes from being buckled in a car seat; it requires work to understand that french fries and mashed potatoes both start out as the same vegetable.)

    2.   Exploring real objects: the child needs to feel, eat, and smell a real orange, for example, not play with a plastic one or a citrus smelly sticker.

C.   Orientation and mobility

    1.   The child needs training to move safely and independently.

    2.   The child requires training to be aware of his/her body position in space.

VIII.   Special care needs

A.   Materials

    1.   Fluorescent-colored dishes, toys, gloves, and socks

    2.   Black felt or blanket close to face level to place materials that will enhance contrast

    3.   Bright, shiny, metallic materials, prisms, color-capped flashlights

    4.   Objects that make noise or move when self-activated (for example, switch toys, simple keyboard, squeak toys, busy boxes, electronic-voice, octagonal roller ball)

5.   Vibrators and vibrating toys, pillows

6.   Firm textures, wood, leather, rubber, beeswax, rocks, balloon filled with water

7.   Temperatures: warm water bottles, plastic ice cube mold, water play, popsicles

8.   Graspable items: hair curlers, tubes, wands, twinkling tube lights, people's fingers, crinkly paper

B.   Control amount of light to avoid glare; glare and shadows impede use of functional vision to see shapes, outlines, movement.

C.   Orient the child thoroughly and systematically to the setting before beginning a new program or changing learning environments.

D.   Clear traffic patterns

1.   Use well-defined, simple spaces (examples: fluorescent masking tape to mark area boundary for block building; carpet squares for circle time).

2.   Ensure safety by keeping doors all the way open or shut; waste cans under tables; chairs pushed under tables.

E.   Display materials at touch- and eye-level.

F.   Adapt picture and print labels to texture signs (example: velcro shape to identify the child's cubby space).

G.   Allow extra time for the child to prepare, begin, and finish each activity.

H.   Peer friendships and assistance

1.   Ask the child's peers to talk more when playing with the child.

2.   Call the child by name when first talking to him/her.

3.   Name objects for child while playing.

4.   Help child "do it for yourself"; don't do it for him/her.

I.   Sequence activities, and provide consistent routines

J.   Physical cuing and guidance for modeling new learning

    1.   Move the child through an activity, fading out structure as the child is able to do more for himself/herself.

    2.   Provide hand-over-hand learning as the child adapts to structured intervention.

    3.   Never grab a child's hands without asking or cuing him/her.

K.   Teaching and using colors

    1.   Many children with visual impairment can discriminate at least primary colors.

    2.   Red is the first color discriminated and easiest to see.

L.   Simple print or painted pictures

    1.   Avoid photographs and magazine pictures, as they are hardest to see.

    2.   Outline important features with thick, black felt pens.

M.   Let children hold objects close, and allow odd head and body postures.

N.   Concrete, real experiences

    1.   Do not overdo use of music tapes and electronic sound toys; sing and provide simple instruments and noisemakers.

    2.   Use materials with weight, texture, temperature; avoid plastic models, blocks, and the like as they have too much "sameness."

    3.   Use the real object whenever possible (example: real food items instead of plastic food items).

O.   Activity changes and transitions

    1.   Say "last turn" or "one more time."

2. Tell and, if needed, use tactile object (one with identifiable features by touch) as preparation for next activity.

P. Active involvement

1. Ask the child to listen quietly to the activity at first, to become curious enough to want to participate.

2. Model the activity by doing it alongside the child.

Q. Possible mannerisms when a child is left alone too long with nothing to do or when stressed

1. The child may engage in body rocking, eye-poking, hand-flicking, or self-stimulating noises without being aware of it.

2. The child should be redirected to a suitable activity — rocking chair or horse, or handed a substitute such as a rattle or music box.

IX. **Responsibilities of caregiver**

A. Ensure the child's safety.

B. Encourage the child's participation, adapting as necessary.

C. Parents/guardians

1. Inspire parents'/guardians' enjoyment and care of child.

2. Promote parents'/guardians' emotional readiness and acceptance of educational and medical intervention, therapies, and public systems.

3. Consider and show acceptance of parents'/guardians' recommendations, visits, and suggestions for the child's care.

4. Make constructive observations, ask questions, and suggest ideas to parents.

BIBLIOGRAPHY

Ferrell, K. A. (1986). *Reach out and teach.* New York: American Foundation for the Blind.

Moore, S. (1985). *Beginnings.* Louisville, KY: American Printing House for the Blind.

Resources for family-centered intervention for infants, toddlers, and preschoolers who are visually impaired (Vols. 1 and 2). (1992). Logan, UT: HOPE, Inc.

Scott, E., Jan, J., & Freeman, R. (1985). *Can't your child see?* Baltimore: University Park Press.

Smith, A., & Cote, K. (1982). *Look at me: A resource manual for the development of functional vision in multiply impaired children.* Philadelphia: Pennsylvania College of Optometry Press.

Teplin, S. W. (1995). Visual impairment in infants and young children. *Infants and Young Children, 8*(1), 18-51.

RESOURCES

American Foundation for the Blind, 1110 Penn Plaza, Suite 300, New York, NY 10001; (212) 502-7600

- *Parenting Preschoolers:* suggestions for raising young blind and visually impaired children
- *Reach Out and Teach:* materials for parents of visually handicapped and multihandicapped young children (parent handbook, reach book and 7 slide/tapes)
- *Touch the Baby:* Blind and visually impaired children as patients — helping them respond to care
- *Preschool Visual Stimulation: It's More Than a Flashlight*
- *An O & M Primer for Families of Young Children*
- *How to Thrive, Not Just Survive:* A guide to developing independent life skills
- *Show Me How*
- *Simon Says is Not the Only Game*
- *Building Blocks* (book and a video, both available in Spanish)

American Printing House for the Blind, P.O. Box 6085, Louisville, KY 40206; (502) 895-2405

- *Parents and Visually Impaired Infants*
- *Beginnings: A Practical Guide for Parents and Teachers of Visually Impaired Babies*
- Sensory Stimulation Kit
- *Hands On* (functional activities for visually handicapped preschoolers)
- *On the Way to Literacy* (handbook plus several tactile story books)
- Overbrook Early Childhood Parent Education Series

Blind Children's Center, 4120 Marathon Street, Box 2915, Los Angeles, CA 90029

- *Heart to Heart:* parents of blind and partially sighted children talk about their feelings (pamphlet and video)
- *Learning to Play:* common concerns for the preschool visually impaired child
- *Move with Me:* a parent's guide to movement development for visually impaired babies
- *Talk to Me:* a language guide for parents of blind children (in English and Spanish)
- *Talk to Me II:* common concerns (in English and Spanish)
- *Welcome to the World:* toys and activities for the visually impaired infant
- *Dancing Cheek to Cheek*
- *Rolling, Crawling, Walking, Let's Get Moving*

(Some available in Spanish)

Hadley School for the Blind, 700 Elm Street, Winnetka, IL 60093 (resources and parent correspondence courses)

- ReachOut and Teach (American Foundation for the Blind) available free to parents enrolled in correspondence course

HOPE, Inc., Ski-Hi Institute, 809 North 800 East, Logan, UT 84321

- Resources for intervention with infants, toddlers, and preschoolers who have visual impairments

ADAPTING LEARNING ACTIVITIES FOR CHILDREN WITH PHYSICIAL/SENSORY IMPAIRMENTS

I. **Overview**

    A.   Work with the parents/guardians and other family members.

        1.   Have parents/family members share their goals for the child in the child care setting.

        2.   Elicit information from parents/guardians and the family on how to work with the child.

    B.   Work with the child's specialists.

        1.   Be a part of development of the child's IFSP (individual family service plan), IEP (individualized education program), or care plan.

        2.   Integrate therapeutic and educational goals into play and other caregiving activities.

        3.   Engage in a communication system with the child's specialist(s) to ensure appropriate carryover and use of the most up-to-date approaches (such as "back-and-forth" notebooks and regular phone calls).

    C.   Integrate children into the whole range of daily activities.

        1.   Plan for their meaningful participation.

        2.   Know the individual child's strengths as well as needs.

        3.   Modify or adapt activities or materials only if the child cannot participate in a meaningful way.

    D.   Learn about and use the child's adaptive equipment/assistive technology.

        1.   Learn the correct use of the child's adaptive equipment (such as hearing aids, communication devices, seating devices).

        2.   Check equipment regularly to be sure that it is working.

        3.   Work with parents/guardians and specialists to develop low-cost alternatives to specialized equipment if necessary (such as special grips for utensils and toys, positioning devices).

E.   Break down daily activities.

    1.   Analyze typical activities to see what skills are necessary for participation; this can help you determine why a child may be having difficulty.

    2.   Provide assistance or adapt activities when needed.

    3.   Pace activities to accommodate the individual child's needs for extra time or quiet time.

F.   Encourage self-confidence and independence.

II.   Adapting the learning environment

A.   Indoor areas

    1.   Measures to ensure access to materials and areas of the room:

        a.   Widen pathways and entrances to activity areas.
        b.   Use tables that accommodate special chairs (or use trays).
        c.   Be sure floors and floor coverings allow a child with a wheelchair or walker to move from place to place.
        d.   Keep toys in sight and within reach; use additional visual or auditory cues if needed.
        e.   Introduce the child to areas of the room verbally or through touch, or both.
        f.   Locate special equipment so the child is still part of the group.
        g.   Remove visual barriers so children can use whatever vision they have to explore the classroom.

    2.   Measures to ensure safety:

        a.   Fasten carpeting securely.
        b.   Keep an eye out for sensory materials (such as play dough, sand, water, shaving cream, finger paints) spilling on the floor.
        c.   Provide protection from sharp corners on furniture.
        d.   Have sturdy furniture for children who use it to support themselves.
        e.   Ensure safety without being overprotective.

3.   Measures to keep the physical environment reasonably constant:

    a.   Keep furniture in the same place from day to day.

    b.   Alert the child to new arrangements verbally or through touch, or both.

    c.   Use different surfaces or floor coverings to help the child organize the physical environment.

B.   Outdoor areas

1.   Consider the outdoor play space an extension of the classroom learning environment.

2.   Provide access to the outdoor space and the equipment.

3.   Ensure safety without being overprotective.

4.   Look at adaptive playground catalogs, and talk with parent/guardian and the child's specialists about possible ways to make the outdoors accessible and safe for the child.

III.   Planning and adapting activities

A.   Know and use the child's communication system (such as sign language, pictures, gestures).

B.   Plan learning activities

1.   Be sure that any modifications allow activities to be as rich and meaningful as those available for peers.

2.   Allow enough time and flexibility in scheduling.

3.   Give verbal and physical assistance cues to supplement environmental cues.

    a.   Position yourself so the child can see your face.
    b.   Speak slowly but not unnaturally.
    c.   Repeat directions in a slightly different way.
    d.   Position the child so the child can see (the caregiver and other children) and do the activity.

4.   Use the least amount of special assistance possible.

       a.   Gently talk or move the child through new activities.

       b.   Encourage the child to watch and listen to the other children.

       c.   Encourage children to help each other.

       d.   If the activity seems too difficult, help the child participate in another way that has the same effect.

       e.   Use open-ended activities (those that allow participation and learning in a variety of ways).

C.   Utilize routines wisely.

    1.   Consider daily routines such as greeting, snack, diapering, and toileting as potential learning times.

    2.   Integrate therapy and educational goals.

    3.   Adapt routines as needed, but don't promote dependence, and don't call extra attention to the child.

    4.   Allow the child enough time.

    5.   Recognize that some children require more assistance and time to complete some self-care routines. Plan for ways to deploy staff efficiently.

    6.   Answer children's questions about special needs honestly and succinctly.

D.   Transitions

    1.   Recognize that transitions may be especially difficult for some children.

    2.   Keep the schedule reasonably consistent.

    3.   Alert children to upcoming transitions.

    4.   Allow time for children to finish what they are doing.

    5.   Remind children and repeat what the next activity will be.

    6.   Plan for children who will be a little early or a little late in making the transitions.

7. Use transition cues that children can attend to and understand (for example, bell, light, verbal direction, picture schedule, sign).

IV. **Selecting and adapting toys and materials**

A. Selecting

1. Use toys and materials that are individually appropriate and age-appropriate.

2. Provide toys and materials that have a wide range of uses and responses.

3. Provide some toys that do not require much manual dexterity.

4. Provide toys that capture the child's interest through sound, sight, touch, or complexity.

5. Include some toys that do not require a lot of strength.

6. Provide some toys and materials that require minimal movements to produce effects.

B. Enlarging

1. Use larger versions of toys or materials.

2. Enlarge essential parts to enhance manipulation; for example, enlarge or emphasize a "button" or switch.

3. Build up handles to enhance grasp.

    a. Wrap handle with foam and tape.
    b. Use a foam hair curler to enlarge the handle.
    c. Use commercially available grips.
    d. Add knobs to puzzles.
    e. Tie a ring to the end of a pull-toy string.

4. Use adaptive scissors, spoons, and the like as needed.

C. Stabilizing

1. Attach play materials to steady the surface, using tape, velcro, C-clamps, and the like.

2. Use magnetic toys.

3.   Attach bells to wrist or ankles.

4.   Use a plastic tray or a cardboard box lid to enclose art supplies or other activity that may get away from children.

5.   Use suction devices such as suction cups, bathtub mats, tacky or adhesive material.

D.   Auditory, visual, and tactile interest

1.   Add or enhance cues to make a toy interesting and meaningful.

2.   Use bright colors, high-contrast colors, and shiny materials.

3.   Use cause-and-effect toys that produce lighted or movement effects as well as sounds.

4.   Use toys of different shapes, textures, and pliability; use texture cues to draw the child's attention to "buttons" or switches.

5.   Be aware of sensory clutter that may distract a child.

6.   Control environmental light and sound to help the child focus and maintain attention.

E.   Positioning for play

1.   If the child is sitting, be sure the child has adequate head and trunk control and, therefore, can use the hands more easily.

2.   Try side-lying as a position for playing on the floor.

3.   Use homemade equipment that serves the purpose and allows the child to be a part of the group. For example, a beanbag chair in the book corner may be appropriate for a child who needs a special seat.

4.   If the child is lying on his/her back, provide shoulder support so he/she can bring up the arms and hands to play.

5. If the child is lying on his/her tummy, place a wedge or bolster underneath so the child's head is up. This allows the child to see and positions arms forward for play.

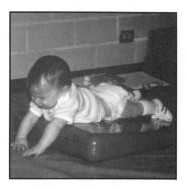

Wedge

6. Mount some materials to the wall instead of using a table surface if that will enhance the child's involvement.

7. Try to keep the child at the same physical level as the other children. For example, if children sit on the floor for music, a child shouldn't be in wheelchair but, instead, on the floor with the rest of the children.

V. Promoting social skills

A. Provide toys that are conducive to social play (such as blocks, dolls, outdoor equipment).

B. Be sure children are close enough together.

C. Permit isolated and onlooker play when indicated.

1. Realize that some children may increase their self-stimulatory behaviors when they are unoccupied.

2. Help children stay engaged in play activities.

D. Stay close enough to children to facilitate play, but not so close as to be distracting.

BIBLIOGRAPHY

Fewell, R. R., & Sandall S. R. (1983). Curricula adaptations for young children: Visually impaired, hearing impaired, and physically impaired. *Topics in Early Childhood Special Education, 2*(4), 51-66.

McCormick, L., & Feeney, S. (1995). Modifying and expanding activities for children with disabilities. *Young Children, 50*(4), 10-18.

Musselwhite, C. (1986). *Adaptive play for special needs children.* San Diego: College Hill Press.

RESOURCES

National Parent Network on Disabilities (Toys tested by Toy Tips®): (414) 288-3386

DOWN SYNDROME

I. Definition and description

A. Down syndrome is one of the most common genetic disorders.

    1. The child is born with an extra chromosome or extra part of a chromosome (21st pair).

    2. The impact of the extra chromosome varies with individuals.

    3. Children with Down syndrome have varying degrees of mental retardation ranging from near normal to severe retardation.

B. Development follows a pattern similar to other children but with delays in reaching milestones.

    1. Early intervention influences early development and later functioning.

    2. The young child tends to show the greatest delays in motor and language development.

    3. Many individuals with Down syndrome will live independently or semi-independently as adults.

II. Incidence: Estimated 1 in 800 to 1 in 1,000 live births.[1]

III. Common physical characteristics (individuals with Down syndrome may or may not have all of these characteristics

A. Facial

    1. Eyes slanted upward

    2. Small fold of skin at inner corners of eyes (epicanthal folds)

---

[1] Incidence figures were provided by Frank Murphy, Executive Director, National Down Syndrome Congress (personal communication, August 3, 1995).

   3.   Small nose and flat bridge of nose

   4.   Protruding tongue

B.   Ears: smaller ears and ear canals

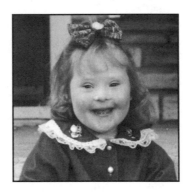

Child with Down syndrome

C.   Hands and feet

   1.   Short and broad hands, with shorter fingers

   2.   Crease across palm (Simian crease)

   3.   Gap between first and second toes

D.   Poor muscle tone ("floppy" baby)

E.   Short stature

IV.   Potential health problems

A.   Congenital heart disease

   1.   More than 40% of children with Down syndrome have some type of heart defect, which is treated with surgery or medications, or both.

   2.   Some young children with heart disease tire more easily than other children during feeding or play.

B.   Intestinal problems

   1.   Possible malformations of the gastrointestinal tract

   2.   Constipation

    C.   Frequent respiratory problems

        1.   Middle-ear infections

        2.   Pneumonia

    D.   Visual problems

        1.   Strabismus (crossed or misaligned eyes)

        2.   Cataracts

        3.   Refractive problems (nearsighted or farsighted)

    E.   Hearing problems: higher risk for hearing loss

    F.   Thyroid problems

    G.   Leukemia

    H.   Muscle/bone problems

        1.   Unstable joints

        2.   Unstable upper spine

V.   Developmental delays

    A.   Extent of delay varies widely from child to child. Table 1 shows the range of developmental markers in children with Down syndrome.

    B.   Social and emotional development may be less delayed than other domains during infancy.

    C.   An individual child's ultimate level of ability is difficult to predict.

VI.   Special care needs

    A.   Infants

        1.   Infant may be difficult to handle because of poor muscle tone.

            a.   Wrap the baby tightly in a blanket to make him/her easier to hold.

b.   Incorporate the holding techniques and exercises recommended by the child's therapists.

c.   Change the infant's position frequently, but encourage voluntary movement and active learning.

Table 1
Developmental Markers for Children
with Down Syndrome

Developmental Marker	Average	Range (in months)
Motor		
Sits	9 months	6 - 16
Pulls to stand	15 months	8 - 26
Walks	19 months	13 - 48
Social/Emotional		
Smiles when talked to	2 months	1½ - 4
Smiles spontaneously	3 months	2 - 6
Recognizes parent	3½ months	3 - 6
Plays pat-a-cake and peek-a-boo	11 months	9 - 16
Self-Help		
Takes solids	8 months	5 - 18
Eats with fingers	10 months	6 - 14
Drinks from open cup	20 months	12 - 30
Is toilet trained (daytime)	36 months	18 - 50
Language		
Speaks first word	18 months	--
Says two words together	30 months	18 - 60

Adapted by permission from Marcel Dekker, publisher of *"The Development of the Child with Down Syndrome: Implications for Effective Education,"* by S. Buckley, in *Medical Care in Down Syndrome: A Preventive Medicine Approach,* edited by P. T. Rogers and M. Coleman (New York: Marcel Dekker, 1992).

---

2.   Feed the infant slowly, with rest periods during feeding. (This is especially important if the infant has a congenital heart defect.)

a. Hold the infant with his/her head slightly raised.

b. When feeding the infant with a spoon, use feeding techniques that encourage lip closure.

c. Be aware of the child's need for more fiber and fluid in the diet.

d. When the child is ready for solid foods, place bits of food on one side of mouth or the other to encourage proper chewing.

3. Early stimulation of all senses is important.

a. Create a nurturing and stimulating environment

b. Be alert to the infant's responses; don't overstimulate.

c. Talk to the infant frequently.

d. Smile, coo, babble.

e. Provide toys at eye level and toys the child can move.

4. To meet the infant's general needs:

a. Interact with the infant rather than do things to or at the infant.

b. Encourage the infant to take turns.

c. Allow the infant enough time to act.

d. Respond to the infant's attempts to interact.

B. Toddlers

1. Developmental delays may be more noticeable at this age.

a. Incorporate suggestions from therapists or specialists.

b. Encourage active play.

c. Help the child learn self-help skills.

d. Encourage normal patterns of creeping/ crawling.

e. Allow the child enough time and opportunity to engage in new activities.

2. Speech and language

a. Encourage regular hearing checks.

b. Be aware of the child's propensity for ear infections and let parent/guardian know if you suspect this in the child.

c. Be aware that some children may require

hearing aids.

d.   Help the child to express himself/herself verbally.

e.   If the child is learning sign language, learn and use it in the care setting.

3.   Dental issues

    a.   Be aware that children with Down syndrome may get their teeth later than other children, and in a different order.

    b.   Encourage good dental care and hygiene.

4.   Obesity (short stature is common and tends to accentuate weight problems)

    a.   Be sure to follow any special dietary guidelines provided (diet should include a lot of fluids and fiber).

    b.   Encourage movement (running and playing active games).

    c.   During play, be aware of the child's tendency for instability of the spinal column.

5.   Plastic surgery to make facial features appear more regular is being debated, with conflicting reports.

C.   Preschoolers

1.   Delayed development is becoming more noticeable.

    a.   Self-help skills

        (1)   Help the child learn to be as independent as possible in self-help skills. Allow time and practice.

        (2)   Be aware that by age 5 most children with Down syndrome feed themselves, take their clothes on and off, run and play, and are toilet-trained during the day.

    b.   Uneven development (social skills may be ahead of cognitive skills)

    c.   Memory and understanding

        (1)   Give specific, clear instructions.

        (2)   Keep requests simple, and check to be sure the child understands.

(3) Repeat statements and requests as often as necessary.

(4) Be a careful observer, and present activities that provide the right amount of challenge.

d. Work with the child's family and team to incorporate the IEP/IFSP goals and objectives within the care setting.

e. Use computers, if available, as educational tools.

2. Children with Down syndrome need guidance techniques similar to those used with their peers, keeping in mind that "difficult" behaviors may appear at a later age and may last longer in children who have Down syndrome.

a. Consider acting-out and other inappropriate behaviors as a frustrated child's attempt to communicate. Respond to the child's intent, but help the child learn more acceptable ways to communicate.

b. Help the child use words to express feelings and needs.

c. Work with all caregivers to keep techniques for guidance and discipline consistent.

d. Suggest a medical evaluation if the child's behavior changes dramatically.

3. Peer interaction

a. Include children in activities and settings with children who do not have disabilities.

b. Help the child learn to play with peers, because this has a positive effect on social development.

c. Help the peers learn how to play with and include the child with Down syndrome.

d. Encourage the child with Down syndrome to participate actively rather than simply observe (the tendency).

4. Children with Down syndrome tend to make immature judgments, their behavior may be impulsive, and they may be more trusting and less aware of potential dangers than other children.

a. Provide more supervision in risky situations (such as crossing streets, dealing with strangers, and so forth.)

      b.   Teach personal safety skills to all children.

VII. Effects on the family

    A.   After receiving the diagnosis of Down syndrome, parents may show signs of grief and loss.

    B.   Support (social, emotional, informational) should be available to the whole family.

    C.   Early intervention and early education programs may have family support programs.

VIII. Questions to ask before caring for child

    A.   Does the child have any major medical/health problems?

        1.   Heart disease

        2.   Intestinal problems

        3.   Respiratory problems

        4.   Hearing or vision problems

    B.   What are the child's developmental needs?

        1.   How does the child communicate?

        2.   What is the child's level of self-care skills?

        3.   What developmental tasks are being worked on in the child's educational or therapy program? Can these be incorporated into the care setting?

        4.   What are the child's favorite activities and toys?

    C.   Any other special concerns?

        1.   Does the child have special feeding needs?

        2.   Does the child need special handling or positioning?

        3.   What therapy and exercises are recommended?

        4.   Does the child have any restrictions on activity?

    D.   How can we provide consistent and coordinated care?

1.   What guidance and disciplinary techniques are being used with the child?

2.   What are the best ways to communicate with the family and with the child's specialized service providers?

BIBLIOGRAPHY

Hanson, M. J. (1987). *Teaching the infant with Down syndrome: A guide for parents and professionals* (2d ed.). Austin, TX: ProEd.

Oeelwein, P. L. (1995). *Teaching reading to children with Down syndrome: A guide for parents and teachers.* Bethesda, MD: New York: Woodbine House.

Rynders, J. E., & Horrobin, J. M. (1995). *Down syndrome: Birth to adulthood.* Denver: Love.

Stray-Gunderson, K. (Ed.). (1995). *Babies with Down syndrome: A new parents guide.* Kensington, MD: Woodbine House.

RESOURCES

National Down Syndrome Congress, 1800 Dempster Street, Park Ridge, FL 60068-1146; 1-800-232-6372

National Down Syndrome Society, 666 Broadway, Suite 810, New York, NY 10012; 1-800-221-4602

MENTAL RETARDATION

I.   **Definition**[1]

    A.   The defining characteristic of mental retardation is substantial limitation in a person's functioning.

        1.   Intellectual functioning well below average.

        2.   Related limitations in two or more adaptive skills areas (skills required to meet the daily demands of diverse community settings).

        3.   Manifested before age 18.

II. **Causes of mental retardation.** In most instances the cause is unknown. Conditions that are known to contribute to mental retardation are:

    A.   Metabolic disorders

        1.   Some disorders cannot be treated and result in mental retardation.

        2.   Some disorders can be treated. If those disorders are detected and treated early, mental retardation can be avoided (for example, PKU).

    B.   Chromosome and other abnormalities such as Down syndrome

    C.   Exposure of the fetus during pregnancy to:

        1.   Substance abuse by the mother (alcohol and other drugs).

        2.   Certain medications used by the mother.

        3.   Infections, such as rubella (German measles) in the mother.

---

[1] Source: American Association on Mental Retardation, *Mental Retardation: Definition, Classification, and Systems and Support,* by Margaret M. Seiter (Ed.) (Washington, DC: American Association of Mental Retardation, 1992).

4.   Extreme levels of radiation.

5.   Underlying illness in the mother, such as heart disease.

D.   Complications of prematurity/low birth weight

E.   Birth trauma

F.   Environmental and social problems (some of these are preventable causes of mental retardation)

1.   Infection

a.   Meningitis (inflammation of the membranes surrounding the brain or spinal cord)
b.   Encephalitis (inflammation of the brain)
c.   Sepsis (presence of pus-forming or other organisms that cause disease)

2.   Trauma

a.   Automobile accidents
b.   Child abuse
c.   Falls

3.   Lack of oxygen

a.   Near drowning
b.   Accidental suffocation

4.   Environmental toxins

a.   Lead poisoning
b.   Carbon monoxide poisoning
c.   Overdose/ingestion poisoning

5.   Social deprivation (low socioeconomic levels and lack of environmental stimulation are linked to mild mental retardation in some cases)

III.   Diagnosis

A.   Important changes are taking place in the ways mental retardation is viewed and assessed.

1.   Diagnosis has been based mainly on IQ and achievement test results.

2.   Now diagnosis also is taking into account the individual's functioning and adaptive skills.

3.   Current assessment trends are focusing on environments and supports that may influence a child's abilities.

4.   Mental retardation is a medical diagnosis that may or may not be accompanied by an additional medical diagnosis.

   a.   Diagnosis may provide information on whether the mental retardation is stable or may worsen.
   b.   One or more conditions in addition to mental retardation may complicate the child's care or response to treatment.
   c.   The younger the child is, the less reliable diagnosis and prognosis are.   A child may achieve a higher level of functioning than expected solely on the basis of diagnosis.

B.   Implications of diagnosis

1.   Use of terms

   a.   The term *developmental delay* is used mostly with infants and toddlers, but sometimes is applied to children older than age 3.
   b.   The term *mental retardation* is applied to some young children with developmental delays. By school age, however, some families may not have been exposed to the term "mental retardation" in connection with their child, even though the child may test as having mental retardation.

2.   Mental retardation means that an individual has difficulty solving problems and organizing tasks that require thinking skills.

3.   Developmental delays may be noticeable in infancy, but the term "mental retardation" generally is not used with children under 3 years of age.

4.   A child should be assessed several different times before being labeled as having "mental retardation."

5.   Not all children who are diagnosed as having development delays before age 3 will be diagnosed as having mental retardation when they are older.

6.   Mental retardation is different from a learning disability (a learning disability refers to a discrepancy between cognitive ability and achievement.)[2]

7.   Children who have mental retardation usually develop in the same general way as other children but at a slower pace. They may not achieve the same level of functioning as children who do not have mental retardation.

IV.   **Categories of mental retardation[3]**

A.   Mild

1.   Most (about 85%) of people diagnosed as having mental retardation are in the mild range, reaching a mental age of 8-12 years old.

2.   They are able to care for their own needs, hold jobs, make friends, and perform skills such as reading, driving, and using a checkbook. They may need special vocational training.

3.   They may show the following developmental delays during early childhood:

a.   Minor lags in walking, talking, self-care during infancy and toddlerhood.

b.   Delays in talking, concept development, and problem-solving during preschool years.

---

[2] The instructor must be able to differentiate mental retardation and learning disability. This may be an issue in states that allow the category "learning disability" for preschool-age children with significant global cognitive delays.

[3] Descriptions of the categories are based on observations of large groups of individuals with mental retardation. Any individual may exceed the level of achievement described for these categories.

4.   Young children will be able to participate in typical early childhood activities such as dramatic play, being read to while looking at books, and playing on playground equipment.

B.   Moderate

1.   Approximately 10% of people diagnosed as having mental retardation are in the moderate range, reaching a mental age of 3-7 years.

2.   These children have noticeable developmental delays, especially in speech, concept development, and problem solving.

3.   They can learn a variety of skills such as eating, dressing, matching and sorting, and word recognition. They may need more structure, repetition, and direct teaching than other children.

4.   As adults, people with moderate mental retardation are capable of working under supervision, such as in fast-food restaurants, as custodians, and as factory workers.

5.   Achieving social skills, such as following instructions and cooperating with others, is as important as learning cognitive skills.

C.   Severe

1.   People with severe mental retardation usually reach the mental age of 2 years.

2.   Obvious developmental delays are noticeable in infancy.

3.   These children lack verbal communication and may communicate through gestures. They may understand more than they are able to communicate verbally.

4.   They can learn basic self-care skills.

5.   With training, individuals may learn some work and leisure skills.

D.   Profound

1.   People with profound mental retardation have minimal capacity for functioning.

2.   They need complete care and supervision.

V.   **Effects on the family**

A.   Families have a wide range of emotional responses.

1.   These emotional responses may have a negative impact on the child and on the caregiver at times.

2.   The actual diagnosis, transitions, and other critical events can trigger emotional responses.

B.   Families of children who are developmentally delayed but undiagnosed may be highly frustrated.

C.   Caregivers should be familiar with community resources, because referrals to infant, toddler, and preschool programs and to parent support programs can offer informational and emotional support to the family.

VI.   **Planning**

A.   Many factors influence the child's ultimate functioning level.

B.   Comprehensive child assessment is needed for planning early education and care.

C.   Setting appropriate and realistic goals and expectations is essential.

D.   An individualized plan (IEP or IFSP) must be developed with a team that includes the family and service providers.

VII.   **Special care needs**

A.   Because early intervention has a crucial influence on later outcomes, caregivers should participate in the development and implementation of the individualized plan.

B.   Infants and toddlers

    1.   Early stimulation of all senses is important.

        a.   Talk a lot to the infant/toddler.
        b.   Be alert to the child's responses; do not overstimulate.
        c.   Use toys that will encourage responses and interaction.
        d.   Encourage the infant/toddler to initiate and take turns in interactions.

    2.   Find out if other intervention strategies are being used.

    3.   Find out what self-feeding techniques are being taught.

C.   Preschoolers

    1.   Adjust your approach to meet the child's developmental or thinking level rather than chronological age.

    2.   Teach and give directions by using simple words. Break down tasks into individual components, and use one-step directions.

        a.   Introduce basic ideas instead of abstract ideas.
        b.   Have children master steps one at a time rather than trying to do a task with many steps all at once.
        c.   Demonstrate at the same time as you give verbal instructions.
        d.   Eliminate distractions.
        e.   Praise the child's efforts as well as successes.
        f.   As the child masters harder tasks or more complex instructions, include these routinely in your interactions with the child.
        g.   Provide many opportunities for the child to practice.

    3.   Motivate the child to learn.

        a.   Use positive reinforcement (reward) that is meaningful and follows naturally from the child's behavior or activity.
        b.   Provide toys, games, and activities that allow the child to feel a sense of accomplishment.

    c.   Find ways to enhance the child's self-esteem.

    d.   Be aware of threats to the child's self-esteem, such as teasing by peers and frustration when unable to keep up with peers.

    e.   Adapt toys as needed. (Examples: enlarge small pieces, stabilize them on a surface, simplify games.)

4.   Provide many experiences and opportunities for active play, learning, and exercise.

    a.   Encourage active learning rather than passive observation (do rather than watch).

    b.   Promote participation and interaction with peers.

    c.   Involve the child in physical activities that match the child's level of development.

5.   Teach and encourage self-care skills, checking with parents/guardians or therapists for specific interventions being used.

6.   Behavior and guidance

    a.   Recognize that children with mental retardation and developmental delays, like all children, sometimes require guidance or discipline.

    b.   Use the same guidance and discipline techniques for similar problem behaviors, whether the child does or does not have mental retardation.

    c.   Expect behaviors in children with mental retardation to appear later chronologically and last longer. (For example, a child with mental retardation who is age 5 may behave more like a child without mental retardation age 3.)

    d.   Help the child find words that express his/her feelings and needs instead of acting out or using other unacceptable behaviors.

    e.   Work with parent/guardian to establish consistent techniques for guidance and discipline.

    f.   Suggest medical evaluation if the child has a dramatic behavior change.

    g.   Maintain consistency and predictability in helping the child learn desirable social behaviors.

    h.   Strive to maintain a pleasant emotional climate.

    7.   Play and peer interactions

        a.   Encourage social behaviors such as getting along with others and making friendships.
        b.   Provide group activities that include the child with mental retardation.
        c.   Model interactions that promote acceptance of all children.

    8.   Safety

        a.   Teach personal safety skills.
        b.   Provide several learning opportunities for children who learn new skills more slowly.
        c.   Supervise children with mental retardation or developmental delays, recognizing that they tend to

            (1)   make immature judgments,
            (2)   behave impulsively, and
            (3)   be more trusting and unaware of potential dangers.

    9.   Provide all children with warmth, nurturance, cuddling, and a responsive physical and social environment.

D.   Health issues

    1.   Encourage early and regular vision and hearing tests.

    2.   Encourage good self-care skills to decrease risks for contagious diseases.

BIBLIOGRAPHY

Allen, K. E., & Schwartz, I. S. (1995). *The exceptional child: Inclusion in early childhood education.* Albany, NY: Delmar.

American Association on Mental Retardation. (1992). *Mental retardation: Definition, classification and systems of support* (9th ed.). Washington, DC: AAMR.

Cohen, H. (1987). Mental retardation. In H. M. Wallace, R. F. Biehl, L. Taft, and A. C. Oglesby (Eds.), *Handicapped children and youth: A comprehensive and clinical approach.* New York: Human Sciences Press.

RESOURCES

The ARC, 500 East Border Street, Third Floor, Arlington, TX 76010; (817) 261-6003

American Association on Mental Retardation, 444 North Capitol Street NW, Suite 846, Washington, DC 20001-1512; 1-800-424-3688 or (202) 387-1968

FETAL ALCOHOL SYNDROME (FAS)

I.   **Definition**

    A.   The diagnosis of fetal alcohol syndrome (FAS) requires the presence of all of these three symptoms:

        1.   Prenatal or postnatal retardation of growth; weight, length, and head circumference are below that of 90% of children.

        2.   A characteristic pattern of facial features.

        3.   Central nervous system damage with resulting neurologic abnormalities, developmental delay, or intellectual impairment, in any combination.

    B.   Children also may have abnormalities in any organ system such as the heart, kidneys, genitals, or bones.

II.   **Incidence**

    A.   In 1993, FAS was reported at a rate of about 6.7 in 10,000 births.[1]

    B.   About 30% - 40% of children born to mothers who drink heavily (five or more drinks per day) have FAS.

    C.   FAS is the most common cause of *preventable* mental retardation.

III.   **Alcohol consumption during pregnancy and breastfeeding**

    A.   Alcohol causes birth defects by changing how cells divide and migrate in the fetus, and, therefore, it affects how the fetus develops.

        1.   There is *no known* safe level of alcohol use during pregnancy.

        2.   In general, more alcohol leads to more problems, although many factors influence the growth and development of the fetus.

---

[1] Source: "Trends in Fetal Alcohol Syndrome" — United States, 1979-1993." *Morbidity and Mortality Weekly Report* (1995, April 7), *44*(13), 249-251.

3.   Pregnant women who drink heavily are more likely to have a miscarriage than those who do not drink.

4.   Women who drink heavily also may lack adequate nutrition and health care, and they are more likely to be using other drugs.

5.   Binge drinking during pregnancy may result in alcohol-related problems for the fetus.

6.   If the mother is breast feeding, alcohol can be passed to the infant in breast milk.

IV.   Common characteristics of children with FAS

A.   Withdrawal

1.   Newborns of mothers who are alcoholic also may be addicted.

2.   When the baby is born or is weaned, exposure to alcohol ceases and the child may go through withdrawal, with any of the following withdrawal symptoms:

a.   Jitteriness
b.   Irritability
c.   Hyperactivity
d.   Cannot be comforted
e.   Difficulty with feeding and sleeping

B.   Growth problems

1.   The newborn's length, weight, and head circumference typically are below what would be expected for that baby's gestational age.

2.   Children continue to be shorter and lighter than their agemates throughout infancy and childhood.

3.   Failure to thrive is a common problem.

C.   Characteristic facial features (children with FAS may not have all of these features)

1.   Small head and flat mid face.

2.   Narrow eye openings, droopy eyes, and small skinfolds (epicanthal fold) at the inner corners of eyes.

3.   Flattened nasal bridge and no groove under nose.

4.   Thin upper lip and small jaw.

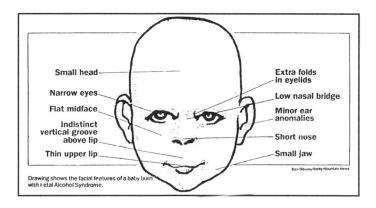

Facial characteristics
Courtesy of Dan Gibson, Rocky Mountain News, Denver, CO

D.   Central nervous system problems

1.   Children with FAS may have a smaller brain. They may show an abnormal brain wave pattern when measured by an electroencephalogram (EEG).

2.   Children are at more risk for intellectual difficulties.

a.   Usually the children with more physical problems also have lower intellectual potential.
b.   Intellectual potential (as measured by a standardized intelligence test) is fairly stable over time. Children with FAS do develop and learn new skills.
c.   Some children who do not have FAS but whose mothers abuse alcohol also may have learning and attention problems that can result in difficulties at school.
d.   Intellectual potential and actual performance levels may not be the same. The environment can support (or limit) a child's performance.

3.   Some newborns have low muscle tone at birth ("floppy" baby). Muscle tone usually improves with age.

4. Developmental delays and symptoms include the following:

    a. During infancy:

        (1) Tremors, seizures.
        (2) Poor motor coordination, poor eye-hand coordination.
        (3) Overly distractable, difficulty adjusting to light, sound, and other sensory input.
        (4) More sensitive to sound than other infants are.
        (5) Poor sucking ability and lack of interest in feeding.
        (6) Difficulty with sleeping.

    b. As the child gets older:

        (1) Poor attention span, slow performance time, hyperactivity.
        (2) Difficulties with speech and language skills.
        (3) Impulsivity, poor reasoning, fearlessness.
        (4) Poor social judgment, difficulty "reading" social cues.
        (5) Overly outgoing, friendly, and inquisitive; may demand a lot of physical contact and affection.
        (6) Difficulty with understanding cause and effect and learning from experiences and mistakes.
        (7) Memory problems.

    c. Individual children may not show all of these characteristics.

E. Associated problems

    1. Skeletal problems such as upper spine abnormalities, joint problems, hip dislocation, abnormalities of feet, toes, fingers, or elbows.

    2. Heart murmurs.

    3. Visual problems.

    4. Ear abnormalities, middle-ear infections, and higher risk for hearing problems.

5.   Cleft lip/palate and other mouth and dental problems.

6.   Genital abnormalities.

7.   Individual children will not show all of these characteristics.

V.   Special care needs and interventions

A.   Overall goal is to help child develop to his/her full potential by providing early mental, emotional, and motor stimulation, as well as communication and coordination with family.

B.   Coordination of plans and services

1.   If the child is eligible for early intervention or special education, the child will have an IFSP (individual family service plan) or IEP (individual education program).

2.   Caregivers should participate in developing the plan so the child's educational and therapeutic goals and objectives can be integrated into the care setting.

C.   Issues related to diagnosis

1.   Children suspected of having FAS need and are entitled to a full diagnostic evaluation by a physician and other specialists.

2.   Early intervention may improve the child's developmental outcome.

3.   Recommended evaluation consists of, but is not limited to:

    a.   Medical evaluation.
    b.   Genetic evaluation.
    c.   Evaluation of language and communication.
    d.   Evaluation of activities of daily living, social skills, and behavior concerns.
    e.   Evaluation of memory, problem solving, achievement, attention, and general intelligence.
    f.   Evaluation of gross and fine motor development.
    g.   Assessment of family resources, needs, and concerns.

D.   Needs and supports for children who are experiencing withdrawal

    1.   Administer medication, if prescribed by a health-care professional.[2]

    2.   Provide a quiet environment with low levels of sensory stimulation.

    3.   Stroke, cuddle, rock, and walk gently as you hold the baby. Watch for the baby's responses to such stimulation.

    4.   Move slowly, gently.

    5.   Follow predictable routines.

    6.   Allow the infant some quiet time without stimulation.

E.   Nutrition issues

    1.   Special concerns of the young child with FAS

        a.   Physical problems can interfere with adequate nutrition.
        b.   Lack of interest in feeding and irritability or distractibility can make feeding times difficult for the child and for the caregiver.
        c.   Older children may not have regular consistent mealtimes.

    2.   Interventions

        a.   When the child is showing withdrawal symptoms or feeding difficulties, a pattern of poor adult-child interaction may begin.

            (1)   Be patient.

---

[2] Administration of medication is generally regarded as an invasive procedure and, as such, is a nursing task that may be subject to statutory provisions or to regulations established by your State's Nursing Board. If this is the case, legislation or regulatory guidelines may be in place that determine whether or not and how this task may be delegated to a non-health-licensed individual (other than the child's parent or guardian). For the safety of the children, and due to the risk of personal and agency liability, you are urged to contact your State Board of Nursing to inquire about the status of delegation of invasive procedures in your state.

        (2)   Provide a consistent and pleasant environment for feeding.

        (3)   Provide rest times within a feeding session to conserve the child's energy.

    b.   Medical or health interventions may be needed.

        (1)   Encourage medical treatment for specific physical problems.

        (2)   Encourage care of the teeth and mouth.

        (3)   Give vitamins,[3] if prescribed by physician.

        (4)   Schedule shorter but more frequent feedings.

        (5)   Give frequent fluids.

        (6)   Keep the infant's head elevated during feedings.

        (7)   Enlarge the bottle nipple's opening so the baby can suck more easily.

F.   Sensory issues

    1.   Special concerns of the child with FAS

        a.   Visual problems include myopia (nearsightedness) and strabismus (crossed eyes).

        b.   Fluid in the ear and middle-ear infections may interfere with hearing.

        c.   FAS children are easily overstimulated by the environment.

    2.   Interventions

        a.   Watch for signs of ear infections.

        b.   Help the family get regular health care.

        c.   Give prescribed medications (follow guidelines for invasive procedures).[4]

        d.   Provide a consistent, structured, and pleasant environment.

        e.   Adjust the amount of sensory stimulation to the level the child can tolerate.

        f.   Use predictable routines.

---

[3] Physician-prescribed vitamins are a medicine, the administration of which should be treated as an invasive procedure in accordance with state regulations.

[4] See footnote 2.

G.   Behavior issues

    1.   Special concerns of the child with FAS

        a.   Difficulty with adapting to new situations, people, and activities.
        b.   Poor social judgment and social skills.
        c.   Difficulty making and keeping friends.
        d.   Head or body rocking.
        e.   Possible problems with eating and sleeping patterns.
        f.   Not easy to comfort.
        g.   Uninhibited and annoying.
        h.   Short attention span for age; highly distractable.
        i.   More challenging behaviors arising from frequent changes in caregivers.

    2. Interventions

        a.   Give children with FAS time, energy, affection, and consistency.

            (1)   Recognize that the provider of child care may be the most consistent person in the child's life.
            (2)   Interact with the infant. Stroke, cuddle, and walk gently with the baby.
            (3)   Be consistent and predictable.
            (4)   Be sure the child understands your instructions and behavioral limits.

        b.   Guide children with FAS toward more appropriate behaviors by organizing the caregiving environment.

            (1)   Set predictable routines and schedules to help the child feel safe and secure and also to foster cognitive development.
            (2)   If possible, have the child with FAS in a smaller group.
            (3)   Create quiet environment with low lighting and noise levels.
            (4)   Break down instructions and activities into small, manageable steps.

c. Adhere to medical interventions, if any; some children may be on medication for hyper-activity or attention problems.[5]

H. Intellectual issues

1. Special concerns for the child with FAS

a. Children with FAS show wide variability in intellectual potential.
b. Short attention span is common.
c. Problems with short-term memory (both visual and verbal memory) are common.

2. Interventions

a. Provide a safe environment.
b. Take precautions to protect the child from injury.
c. Be aware of the child's tolerance level for sensory stimulation (visual, auditory, and touch).
d. Utilize the physical environment to provide consistent play centers, storage spaces, and so forth.
e. Be aware of the child's developmental level in the following interventions:

(1) Use gestures and verbal prompts to help the child focus attention.
(2) Use models to demonstrate the desired behavior, and help the child pay attention to the model.
(3) Plan and use the physical environment to help tell the child about behavioral expectations; try not to overuse verbal directions.
(4) Use visual cues such as pictures, labels, and photographs to help the child gain access to toys and materials, and to return them to their storage space.
(5) Provide a lot of learning opportunities throughout the day so the child has many chances to learn new skills.

---

[5] See footnote 2.

(6)   To encourage appropriate behaviors, provide reinforcement that is linked meaningfully to the child's activity or behavior.

(7)   Avoid abrupt changes in activities; give several cues regarding upcoming transitions.

(8)   Prevent behavior problems by having reasonable expectations for the child's age and developmental level; don't spend too much time in large-group activities, shorten waiting time, spend time in child-initiated, active play.

(9)   Break tasks, activities, and routines into small parts to help the child learn and be more independent.

I.   Motor

1.   Special concerns for the child with FAS

a.   The child may be clumsy.
b.   The child may have poor eye-hand coordination.

2.   Interventions

a.   Implement any occupational and physical therapy recommendations.
b.   Organize the physical environment for accessibility and safety.
c.   To encourage fine motor (small muscle) skills, use magnetic toys and adaptive scissors, spoons, or drawing implements.

J.   Child abuse and neglect

1.   Special concerns of the child with FAS

a.   Children may be at higher risk because of their home environment and their challenging behaviors.
b.   Children may be more at risk if the child lives with the biological mother who continues to drink.
c.   The family may need additional help to deal with child's challenging behaviors.

2.   Interventions

    a.   Be aware of social service reporting requirements for abuse and neglect.

    b.   Provide families with information and referral for respite care.

    c.   Be familiar with the center's policies that define the provider's role if a parent comes to pick up the child and is under the influence of alcohol, fails to pick up the child, is late consistently, or needs reminders to pick up child.

VI.   Caregiver actions

A.   Be aware that the child's difficulties may be rooted in an underlying organic problem.

    1.   Obtain information from a knowledgeable source such as a physician, a health professional, or a child development specialist.

    2.   Encourage the family to have a multidisciplinary evaluation of their child. Follow the referral procedures established by your center.

        a.   Evaluation findings may result in better understanding of the child's physical problems and corresponding behavioral difficulties.

        b.   Evaluation results may lead to treatments and interventions that can reduce or help manage the behavioral difficulties.

        c.   Evaluation results may provide a more realistic picture of the child's current abilities, strengths, and needs.

    3.   Be sure the family is aware that Child Find evaluations are available to families at no cost through the local school district.

    4.   Be an information resource for the family.

B.   Provide a support system for the child within the care setting.

    1.   Individualize curriculum and activities as needed for the child.

    2.   Identify a peer helper for the child.

3.   Focus on helping the child learn functional skills and communication skills.

4.   Be optimistic. Infants and young children with FAS will grow, develop, and learn.

C.   Establish a communication system between the home and the center.

1.   Share effective behavior management techniques with parents to encourage consistency between home and the center.

2.   Try to avoid crises by having an ongoing communication system.

3.   Plan time to talk, use notebooks that go back and forth between home and center, schedule regular phone calls, or whatever method works for an individual family.

D.   Be aware of community resources, share information with families, and encourage their participation for informal social support.

1.   Crisis intervention services.

2.   Mental health services.

3.   Parent support groups.

4.   Teams of professionals who work with the child and family.

5.   Financial assistance.

6.   Early intervention services, Child Find, and other special education services.

7.   Respite care.

8.   Encourage the family's participation in the community for informal social support.

BIBLIOGRAPHY

Dorris, M. (1989). *The broken cord.* New York: Harper Perennial.

Steinmetz, G. (1992). Fetal alcohol syndrome: The preventable tragedy. *National Geographic, 181*(2), 36-39.

Williams, B. F., et al (1994). Fetal alcohol syndrome: Developmental characteristics and directions for future research. *Education and Treatment of Children, 17*(1), 86-97.

RESOURCES

Healthy Mothers, Healthy Babies Coalition, 409-12th Street SW, Washington, DC 20001; (202) 863-2458

March of Dimes, Birth Defects Foundations, 1275 Mamaroneck Avenue, White Plains, NY 10605; (914) 428-7100

National Clearinghouse for Alcohol and Drug Information, P.O. Box 2345, Rockville, MD 20852; (301) 468-2600

National Council on Alcoholism and Drug Dependence (NCADD), Coalition on Alcohol and Drug Dependent Women and Their Children, 1511 K Street NW, Suite 443, Washington, DC 20005; (202) 737-8122

U. S. Public Health Service, Public Affairs Office, Hubert H. Humphrey Bldg., 200 Independence Avenue SW, Room 647-D, Washington, DC 20201; (202) 690-7850

ADAPTING LEARNING FOR CHILDREN WITH COGNITIVE DELAYS

I. **Overview**

   A. Children with, or at risk for, cognitive delays or disabilities are likely to have problems with attention, memory, problem solving, and concept development.

   B. Some (but not all) children with cognitive delays will have delays in other areas of development.

   C. Cognitive and language development are closely related.

   D. Exploration, play, and interaction are to be encouraged.

   E. Children with cognitive delays need many of the same learning activities and methods as other children.

II. **Infants**

   A. Responsive, consistent caregiving

   1. Learn about the individual child and allow the child to learn about you.

   2. Utilize physical positions that are comfortable for the child; increase stroking, cuddling, rocking, and walking with the infant as the infant tolerates such handling.

   3. Talk with the infant.

      a. Smile, coo, babble, and sing.
      b. Create "conversations" or turn-taking exchanges.
      c. Give the infant ample time to take a turn (wait).
      d. Encourage the child to initiate some of these "conversations."
      e. Be alert to the infant's responses; don't overstimulate.
      f. Allow some quiet time.

   4. Use social routines, games, and infant activities that encourage interaction.

      a. Play peek-a-boo and similar games.
      b. Introduce books; read with the baby.

    B.   Physical environment

        1.   Provide a quiet environment for infants who need it.

            a.   Be aware of the infant's response to stimulation.
            b.   Increase sensory stimuli gradually as the infant tolerates it.

        2.   Be sure that toys and materials are safe, interesting, and accessible.

            a.   Provide toys that do something when the child shakes, swipes at, or drops them, such as roly-poly toys, rattles, and balls.
            b.   Be sure the child can reach for, look at, listen to, hold, and drop the toys.
            c.   Place toys at the appropriate eye level and distance.
            d.   As the infant becomes stronger and more capable, provide toys that are more challenging.

        3.   Provide consistency in routines. When infants feel secure in their environment, they will do more, communicate more, and become more confident in exploring and learning.

    C.   IFSP (individual family service plan) for infants eligible for Part C services.

        1.   Participate with the parent/guardian and other team members in developing the plan.

        2.   Integrate educational and therapeutic objectives into the child-care setting.

        3.   Use the resources of other members of the IFSP team.

III. Toddlers

    A.   More noticeable developmental delays

        1.   Continue to work with parent/guardian and other team members to integrate the child's educational and therapeutic objectives into the child care setting.

        2.   Provide assistance as needed, but don't overdo.

3. Continue to encourage active play and exploration and interaction with adults and children.

4. Help the child learn self-help skills.

5. Be aware that activities may take longer to complete and require more practice to learn.

B. Support for the toddler's cognitive development

1. Continue to provide predictable routines.

2. Organize the physical environment to direct the child's attention to the play center or other area.

3. Provide many practice opportunities in keeping with the child's interests.

4. If necessary, break down activities or instructions into smaller parts the child can manage.

5. Continue to provide toys that do something when the child acts on them.

    a. Provide "cause-and-effect" toys.
    b. Include some toys that require putting two or more actions together.
    c. Provide toys that encourage symbolic play, such as baby dolls and housekeeping toys.

6. Read books together.

C. Support for the toddler's speech and language development

1. Because ear infections and hearing loss can interfere with speech and language:

    a. Watch for signs of ear infections.
    b. Encourage early and regular hearing tests.

2. Continue the "conversational" approach; encourage the child to make requests, make comments, begin to ask questions, and answer.

3. Respond to the child's attempts to communicate through sounds, gestures, and words; model appropriate language, but don't correct.

4.   If a child uses sign language or another system to communicate, work with the parent/guardian and the child's team to use the same form of communication within the child care setting.

5.   Be aware that a child may understand more language than he/she is able to express.

D.   Support for the toddler's social development

1.   Provide frequent, positive feedback.

2.   Structure the environment (through predictable routines, organized play, and learning centers) to help the child understand the "rules."

3.   Help the child quiet down after vigorous play.

4.   Help (give cues, show) the child play with or near other children in an uncrowded setting; have more than one of a given toy if possible.

5.   Plan for transition times.

a.   Give the child extra cues as to what will happen next.
b.   Try for unhurried transitions.

IV.   Preschoolers

A.   More apparent cognitive delays

1.   Know the individual child, recognizing that children vary widely in cognitive ability.

2.   Realize that a child may show uneven development across developmental domains.

3.   Be aware of children's capabilities and difficulties when planning activities, and plan activities for groups composed of children with a range of ages.

4.   Encourage and teach self-care skills.

a.   Consult with the child's specialists about specific methods.
b.   Break self-care skills into small parts for teaching.
c.   Provide lots of practice.

B. IEP (individualized education program) for preschoolers eligible for special education

   1. Participate with parent/guardian and team members in developing the plan.

   2. Integrate goals and objectives into the child-care setting.

   3. Use the resources of the other team members.

C. Support for the preschooler's cognitive development

   1. Keep directions simple.

   2. Use forms of assistance that help the individual child.

      a. Modeling (by adult or peer)
      b. Gestures
      c. Repeating directions
      d. Visual cues (pictures, labels, and the like)
      e. Physical assistance
      f. Working with a peer

   3. Sequence learning activities into small steps, but be sure the child experiences the whole activity; activities should be meaningful.

   4. Allow enough time to try, practice, and repeat.

   5. Give positive reinforcement that is genuine and is linked naturally to the child's behavior or activity.

   6. Continue to utilize the physical environment to support learning.

   7. Assist the child with fine-motor activities or playing with toys, if needed.

   8. Make adaptations by stabilizing or enlarging, as needed.

   9. Link the various experiences and activities to reinforce memory (for example, talk about and do activities related to field trips).

10.   Create a "literacy-rich environment." Read books and use *environmental print* (maximize reading opportunities by labeling play areas, using menus and posting simple signs).

D.   Support for the preschooler's speech and language development

1.   Encourage communication, and give the child ample time to communicate.

2.   Work with any specialists the child has.

3.   If the child uses an augmentative communication system (sign language, pictures, computer), also use it in the child care setting.

4.   If the child has articulation difficulties, listen carefully. Most children have consistent patterns, and you should be able to understand the child's intent by listening carefully.

5.   Expand on what the child says.

6.   Talk about what you are doing and what the other children are doing.

7.   Model correct usage and pronunciation instead of correcting.

8.   Explain new concepts and vocabulary using pictures and models.

9.   Help the other children to understand what the child is saying or attempting to say.

E.   Support for the preschooler's social development

1.   Provide activities, toys, and games that allow the child to feel a sense of accomplishment.

2.   Encourage and teach play with peers. Help peers to understand the child, share toys with the child, ask the child to join in play, and so forth.

3.   Be aware that social behaviors more typical of younger children (for example, oppositional behavior) may appear during the preschool years.

F. Behavior and discipline

    1. Keep the same primary caregiver at the center, if possible.

    2. Help children control their own behavior by structuring the environment and defining the space.

    3. Give directions that are simple, sequenced, and organized.

    4. Help children control their own behavior by enforcing the rules.

    5. Provide frequent positive feedback; reinforce sustained and focused attention.

    6. Be aware that a child's speech and language delays may lead to difficulties in expressing wants, needs, and feelings:

        a. Recognizing that "acting out" may be a child's way of communicating, respond to the child's intent, but help the child learn more appropriate ways of communicating.

        b. Teach children words for expressing their feelings.

    7. Prevent behavior problems when possible.

        a. Redirect the child.
        b. Join the child's play.
        c. Provide a gentle touch to help the child regain control.

    8. Have reasonable expectations for group activities; spend less time in circles and activities that require a lot of sitting, waiting, and watching.

    9. Give children several cues before making the transitions.

G. Safety

    1. Be aware that cognitive delays may lead to immature judgments or seeming lack of awareness in risky situations (for example, around playground equipment).

2.   Expect impulsive behaviors to be more common.

3.   Provide more supervision than for peers of the same age in crossing streets, meeting strangers, and other safety issues, but don't limit the child's opportunities to learn how to deal with risky situations.

4.   Teach personal safety skills to all children, adjusting examples, instructions, and practice opportunities for children with cognitive delays or disabilities.

BIBLIOGRAPHY

Allen, K. E., & Schwartz, I. S. (1995). *The exceptional child: Inclusion in early childhood education*. Albany, NY: Delmar.

Bricker, D., & Cripe, J. J. W. (1992). *An activity-based approach to early intervention*. Baltimore: Paul H. Brookes.

Wolery, M., & Wilbers, J. S. (Eds.) (1994). *Including children with special needs in early childhood programs*. Washington, DC: National Association for the Education of Young Children.

PRENATAL EXPOSURE TO DRUGS

I. **Nature of the problem**

A. The use of drugs (prescribed, over-the-counter [OTC], tobacco, alcohol, or illicit) during pregnancy and breastfeeding can have major health implications for fetal (and postnatal) development.

1. Drugs can cause variations in development and toxic or addictive problems in the fetus.

2. Maternal drug use also may have long-term negative effects on the child's physical, neurologic, and behavioral development, which may affect the child's intelligence and abilities to concentrate and learn.

3. Street drugs, alcohol, and OTC drugs can get into the breast milk and be passed to the infant.

B. Types of drugs. A variety of legal and illegal drugs pose a threat to development of the fetus. These include

1. prescribed medications such as tranquilizers, sleeping medications, drugs for pain or seizure control, and drugs for emotional stress;

2. medications that can be purchased over-the-counter without a prescription;

3. nicotine and alcohol;[1] and

4. illegal drugs such as cocaine, crack, hallucinogens, marijuana, and narcotics.

C. Factors influencing the effect of drug use during pregnancy and delivery include

1. the amount and type of drugs used,

2. when and for how long the drug exposure occurs,

3. the combination of drugs used (including alcohol),

---

[1] The effects of prenatal exposure to alcohol are treated separately in the lesson on fetal alcohol syndrome.

4.   individual maternal and fetal biological sensitivity to drugs, and

5.   prenatal care and maternal nutrition.

D.   The need for drugs often interferes with the addicted mother's self-care and care for her developing child.

II.   Prevalence

A.   Substance exposure rates among pregnant women are difficult to estimate and often are inaccurate. Furthermore, exposure does not necessarily harm the fetus or child.

1.   Estimated rates of exposure vary widely by mother's age, educational level, marital status, and inner-city versus other residential setting.

2.   Few national studies have reflected accurately the ethnic, racial, and economic makeup of U.S. women and infants.

3.   Detection issues

a.   Maternal self-reporting of drug use underestimates exposure because many women are reluctant to say they are doing this.
b.   Blood and urine tests for drugs usually detect only substances used recently and may not be conducted at all if no symptoms are apparent.

B.   An estimated 100,000-375,000 women each year give birth to children prenatally exposed to illicit drugs.[2]

C.   Following are the estimated rates of substance use by pregnant women between ages 12 and 34 years:[3]

1.   Use of cocaine, hallucinogens, sedatives, and stimulants ranges from 1% to 3%.

---

[2] From *Drug-Exposed Infants: A Generation at Risk* (Report to the Chairman, Committee on Finance, U.S. Senate), by the U.S. General Accounting Office, June 28, 1990 (Washington, DC: U.S. Government Printing Office).

[3] From "Estimating the Number of Substance-Exposed Infants," by Deanna S. Gomby & Patricia H. Shiono, 1991, in *The Future of Children, 1*(1), 17-25 (a publication of the Center for the Future of Children, the David and Lucille Packard Foundation).

2. Opiate use rates vary dramatically from report to report because of differences in study methods and location.

3. Marijuana usage is estimated to be between 3% and 12%.

4. Estimated alcohol abuse is 3% (73% of women are estimated to drink at some point during the pregnancy).

5. The rate of cigarette smokers is estimated to be 37.6%.

III. Interacting factors

A. Drug users often stress the developing fetus further by using cocaine or other drugs in combination with alcohol or other central nervous system depressants (polydrug abuse).

B. Infant mortality rates are raised by the combined effects of exposure to drugs, poor maternal nutrition, and lack of prenatal care.

C. The roles of prenatal exposure, genetic influence, prematurity, and environmental factors in determining a child's long-term difficulties are *unclear*. Long-term implications of prenatal drug exposure are unknown at this time.

IV. Typical characteristics of children exposed prenatally to drugs

A. Drug withdrawal

1. Drug withdrawal in newborns can be detected during the first 10 days after the last exposure to the drug; effects of withdrawal can last up to 6 months.

2. Symptoms that occur in children exposed prenatally to opiates (methadone, heroin) but not in children exposed prenatally to cocaine include

a. irritability,
b. diarrhea,
c. vomiting,
d. high-pitched cry,
e. continual movement, and
f. ineffective sucking,

B.   Other possible characteristics

1.   During the first 6 weeks of life

a.   Withdrawal symptoms
b.   Unusual wakefulness and irritability
c.   Tremors
d.   High-pitched crying
e.   Sensitivity to light
f.   Increased muscle tone (rigidity)
g.   Poor feeding and weak and ineffective sucking
h.   Difficulty adapting to environmental stimulation
i.   Difficulty becoming or remaining alert
j.   Difficulty with social interaction

2.   Infants (6 weeks to about 1 year of age)

a.   Disturbed sleep and wakefulness patterns
b.   Seemingly unresponsive to routine stimuli (such as voice, touch) but startled easily by sudden changes
c.   Seem to dislike human contact
d.   Arch when held

3.   Toddlers/preschoolers (ages 1-5 years)

a.   Irregular sleep and eating patterns
b.   Difficulties with attachment to primary providers of care
c.   Apathy (disinterested behavior, listlessness)
d.   Delays in reaching age-appropriate play patterns or language/communication skills
e.   Hyperactivity
f.   Delays in fine- and gross-motor skills or excessive awkwardness
g.   Attention problems
h.   Overly sensitive to sound and light

4.   The effects of prenatal exposure to drugs that arise as children reach preschool years are not fully understood yet, although sensitivity to environmental stimulation is likely to persist.

C. Effects associated with use of specific drugs during pregnancy

1. *Cocaine*[4]

   a. Severe bleeding of the placenta
   b. Higher risk of prematurity
   c. Low birth weight
   d. Fetal distress (adverse effects of maternal factors on the fetus)
   e. Insufficient blood supply to the fetus's brain

2. *Opiates*

   a. May have symptoms listed for cocaine
   b. Increased risk of SIDS (sudden infant death syndrome, or "crib death")
   c. Physical, intellectual, perceptual, and behavioral problems

3. *Marijuana*

   a. Small size at birth
   b. Long-term effects are uncertain

4. Smoking *tobacco* during pregnancy

   a. More miscarriages among smoking women
   b. Small size for gestational age (age since conception)

V. **Exposure to drugs after birth**

A. Children should not be exposed to smoke, including smoke in the child care environment. Passive exposure to cigarette smoke, crack, or marijuana smoke may contribute to

1. increases in bronchitis/pneumonia,

2. asthma/wheezing,

3. ear infections, and

4. greater risk for SIDS.

---

[4] Care should be taken to avoid relying on media reports and generalizations regarding prenatal exposure to cocaine.

B.   Drugs may be passed to an infant through breast milk.

VI.   **Special care needs and interventions**. Early intervention may lessen the severity of problems in children exposed prenatally to drugs. When exposure is known or suspected, a full diagnostic evaluation should be conducted to assess physical, behavioral, and cognitive development.

A.   *Nutrition*. Infant feeding problems may be attributable to ineffective sucking, disinterest in feeding, withdrawal symptoms, irritability and hyperactivity, and the need for frequent feeding.

1.   Be sure that feeding schedules and methods are responsive to the child's needs.

2.   If the infant/child is failing to thrive, tube feeding may be necessary.[5]

B.   *Environment*. Because of maternal drug use and drug-seeking, the child may experience environmental deprivation, neglect or abuse, abandonment, unpredictable care, drugs in breast milk, or placement in foster care.

1.   Be patient, and try to have compassion for these children and their families.

2.   Encourage bonding between the child and care providers.

3.   Provide a safe, predictable, and nurturing environment for the child.

4.   Provide a consistent routine in the child care environment.

5.   Protect the child from injury.

6.   Know your state's child abuse and neglect reporting regulations. Be alert to signs of, and report, suspected abuse or neglect.

---

[5]   Tube feeding (gastrostomy tube feeding or G-tube feeding) is an invasive procedure and, therefore, subject to state regulation in most states. You are urged to contact your state board of nursing so that policies and practices related to invasive procedures are in compliance with the law. These laws stipulate whether such procedures may or may not be performed by non-health licensed individuals, and the terms for delegation and supervision of these tasks.

7. Follow your center's written policy (which should include a contract with the parent) that spells out what you should do if the parent does not come for the child or is under the influence of drugs or alcohol.

8. Refer parent to appropriate community agencies and support groups, as needed.

9. Assist in referral for medical problems.

10. Share information regarding parenting skills.

C. *Neurobehavioral dysfunction*

1. Symptoms may include

    a. lethargy;
    b. irritability;
    c. poor response to faces/voices;
    d. inability to follow movement with eyes;
    e. inconsolability;
    f. abnormal reflexes or muscle tone; and
    g. sleep difficulties such as continual motion, crying during sleep, and waking in an irritable or disorganized state.

2. Medications may be prescribed for withdrawal symptoms or seizures.[6]

3. Helpful actions include

    a. lowering light, noise, and activity levels in the environment;
    b. swaddling to comfort infants;
    c. avoiding forced eye contact;
    d. using appropriate positioning to improve physical movements;
    e. using pacifiers as needed;

---

[6] Administration of medication is generally regarded as an invasive procedure and, as such, is a nursing task that may be subject to regulations established by your State's Nursing Board. If this is the case, legislation or regulatory guidelines may be in place that determine whether or not and how this task may be delegated to a non-health-licensed individual (other than the child's parent or guardian). For the safety of the children, and due to the risk of personal and agency liability, you are urged to contact your State Board of Nursing to inquire about the status of delegation of invasive procedures in your state.

f.   avoiding propping bottle;

g.   handling with soothing and gentle touch;

h.   increasing stimulation over time, in response to infant cues;

i.   increasing stroking, cuddling, rocking, massage; and

j.   relying on infant's cues as guidelines for the above, and for pacing all interactions.

VII. Working with the parent

A.   Women of childbearing age who are addicted to drugs face many barriers to good outcomes for themselves and their children, including

1.   legal prosecution and societal indifference or scorn;

2.   failure of professionals to detect or react to parental drug use, especially by middle- and upper-class women;

3.   shortage of drug treatment programs for pregnant women or inability to enter treatment programs for practical reasons (money, child care, or transportation);

4.   the compelling need for drugs that may be stronger than the need for treatment; and

5.   poverty and violence that often are part of a drug-use lifestyle.

B.   When substance abuse is suspected, encourage the mother to

1.   seek medical monitoring for the use of over-the-counter or prescribed medications during pregnancy and breastfeeding;

2.   arrange for prenatal care as soon as possible. Preferably, seek health care prior to pregnancy; and

3.   seek appropriate drug treatment programs or refer her to other appropriate community resources when available.

BIBLIOGRAPHY

Behrman, R. E. (Ed.). (1991). Drug-exposed infants [Special issue]. *The Future of Children, 1*(1).

Rossetti, L. M. (1992). *Developmental problems of drug-exposed infants.* San Diego: Singular Publishing Group.

Sparks, S. N. (1993). *Children of prenatal substance abuse.* San Diego: Singular Publishing Group.

Zuckerman, B., & Brown, E. R. (1993). Maternal substance abuse and infant development. In C. H. Zeanah (Ed.), *Handbook of infant mental health* (pp. 120-142). New York: Guilford Press.

RESOURCES

American Council for Drug Education, 204 Monroe Street, Rockville, MD 20850; 1-800-488-3784

Child Welfare League of America, 440 First Street NW, Suite 310, Washington, DC 20001; (202) 638-2952

Healthy Mothers, Healthy Babies Coalition, 409 12th Street SW, Washington, DC 20024-2188; (202) 863-2458

National Center for Family-Centered Care, Association for the Care of Children's Health, 7910 Woodmont Avenue, Suite 300, Bethesda, MD 20814-3015; (301) 654-6549

National Clearinghouse for Alcohol and Drug Information, P.O. Box 2345, Rockville, MD 20852-2345; 1-800-729-6686 or (301) 468-2600

National Council on Alcoholism and Drug Dependence (NCADD), Coalition on Alcohol and Drug Dependent Women and Their Children, 1511 K Street NW, Suite 443, Washington, DC 20005; (202) 737-8122

National Maternal Child Health Clearinghouse, 8201 Greensboro Drive, Suite 600, McLean, VA 22102; (703) 821-8955, ext. 265

PEDIATRIC HIV INFECTION

I. Definitions

A. *Human immune deficiency virus (HIV):* the infectious agent that causes AIDS.

  1. Individuals are HIV-positive after they are infected with the virus but may or may not yet have symptoms.

  2. Individuals who are HIV-positive can transmit the virus to others under specific circumstances.

  3. Pediatric HIV infection refers to HIV infection occurring in children under the age of 13 years. The infection develops more rapidly and with different symptoms in children than in adults.

B. *Acquired immune deficiency syndrome (AIDS):* a cluster of symptoms developing in a person who is HIV-positive, resulting from severe impairment of the immune system. A diagnosis of AIDS requires the presence of HIV and specific patterns of symptoms.

II. Diagnosis and outlook

A. Exposure to HIV

  1. Most children (about 90%) who get HIV acquire it from their infected mothers before birth or during the birth process.[1]

  2. HIV infection develops in 15% - 30% of children born to mothers who are HIV-infected.[2]

---

[1] "Epidemiology of Pediatric Human Immunodeficiency Virus Infection in the United States," by M. F. Rogers, M. B. Caldwell, M. L. Gwinn, & R. J. Simonds, *Acta Paediatrica (Supplement) 400*, (1994). 5-7.

[2] From *Evaluation and Management of Early HIV Infection*, Clinical Practice Guideline No. 7 (AHCPR Publication no. 94-0572), by W. El-Sadr, J. M. Oleske, B. D. Agins, B. D., et al. (Rockville, MD: Agency for Health Care Policy and Research, Public Health Service, U. S. Department of Health and Human Services, January, 1994).

B.   HIV antibodies (protective substances the body produces to combat the HIV virus) can be detected by a blood test a short time after exposure to HIV.

1.   Infants can carry antibodies acquired from their mothers and later test negative (not infected).

2.   If a child does not have HIV infection, the antibody usually disappears at around 9 months of age, but it may remain as long as 18 months.

3.   At birth, children who themselves have HIV infection cannot be differentiated from those who carry their mothers' antibodies but are not infected.

4.   Continued testing for the virus is essential to determine the need for treatment.

C.   Diagnostic categories for pediatric HIV infection:[3]

1.   Children who are known to have HIV or AIDS

2.   Children who were born to mothers who had the infection but whose own infection status is not yet known

3.   Children who were born to HIV-infected mothers but later test negative (do not have HIV).

D.   Outlook

1.   HIV infection in infants and young children progresses more quickly than in adults, and the symptoms are different.

---

[3]   From 1994 Revised Classification System for Human Immunodeficiency Virus Infection in Children less than 13 Years of Age; Official Authorized Addenda: Human Immunodeficiency Virus Infection Codes and Official Guidelines for Coding and reporting ICD-9-CM, by Centers for Disease Control and prevention, in *Morbidity and Mortality Weekly Report, 43*(RR-12) (Sept. 30, 1994), 1-19.

    2.   By 1 year of age, about a fourth of children with HIV infection will have AIDS.[4] Other children may not show symptoms for several years.

    3.   Life expectancy is not known, although new medications have lengthened the survival time.

III. Impact of HIV infection

    A.   Lowers functioning of the immune system.

    B.   Makes the child more susceptible to infections.

    C.   Increases the risk for getting certain cancers.

    D.   Can infect the central nervous system.

IV. Incidence[5]

    A.   *Pediatric AIDS* cases in the United States

        1.   AIDS is the seventh leading cause of death (and rising) among children ages 1 to 4, as well as for ages 5 through 14 years.[6]

        2.   *Overall*

            a.   Slightly more than 1,000 *new* cases of pediatric AIDS were reported to the Centers for Disease Control and Prevention in 1994.
            b.   By the end of 1994, 6,209 cases of pediatric AIDS had been reported to CDC.
            c.   The actual incidence of AIDS is underreported because of the delay between the diagnosis of AIDS and the time the cases are reported.

---

[4] From "Developmental Issues: Children Infected with the Human Immunodeficiency Virus," by C. B. Johnson, in *Infants and Young Children,* (1993), *6*(1), 1-10.

[5] Incidence figures presented are those reported through December, 1994, in *HIV/AIDS Surveillance Report, 6*(2), by Centers for Disease Control and Prevention, Atlanta.

[6] Advanced Report of Final Mortality Statistics, 1992," by K. D. Kochanek & B. L. Hudson, *Monthly Vital Statistics Report, 43*(6) (supplement) (Hyattsville, MD: National Center for Health Statistics, 1995).

3.   *Racial/ethnic distribution of pediatric AIDS*

    a.   Black children account for 56% of cases (they account for only 15% of the children in the United States).[7]

    b.   Hispanic children account for 24% of cases (they account for only 10% of the children in the United States).[8]

    c.   White children account for 19% of cases.

    d.   American Indian and Alaskan Native children account for less than 1% of cases.

    e.   Asian and Pacific Islander children account for less than 1% of cases.

B.   Reported cases of *pediatric HIV infection* cases (based on information from 21 states)[9] (There is no required national reporting system of children who are infected with HIV who do not have AIDS.)

1.   *Overall*

    a.   For every one child with AIDS, an estimated two additional children have the HIV infection.[10]

    b.   By the end of 1994, more than 1,100 children who did not have AIDS were reported as having HIV infection.

2.   *Racial/ethnic distribution of pediatric AIDS infection*

    a.   Black children account for 57% of cases.

    b.   White children account for 26% of cases.

    c.   Hispanic children account for 12% of cases.

---

[7]   "Epidemiology of Human Immunodeficiency Virus Infection in Children," by A. Willoughby, *Annals of Allergy,* (1994), *72*(3), 185-194.

[8]   See footnote 4.

[9]   Although the figures reported for HIV infection were based on information from 21 states, according to the Centers for Disease Control and Prevention, by December, 1994, 25 states had enacted confidential reporting of confirmed HIV infection (Centers for Disease Control and Prevention, *HIV/AIDS Surveillance Report, 6*(2), (1994).

[10]   See footnote 4.

d. American Indian and Alaskan Native children account for 1% of cases.

e. Asian and Pacific Islander children account for less than 1% of cases.

3. Most children with HIV infection are cared for at home, with periodic clinic visits and hospitalizations.

V. How the disease is contracted

A. *Truths*. HIV is transmitted by three primary means:

1. Sexual contact (semen, vaginal fluids) with a person who has HIV infection

a. Unprotected sexual activities and sexual practices that cause tears in lining of rectum, vagina, penis.

b. Unprotected sexual activities with injecting drug users.

2. Exposure to the blood of a person who has the HIV infection

a. Sharing contaminated needles and syringes by intravenous drug users, or

b. Receiving a transfusion of infected blood or blood products mainly between 1978 and 1985; rare now.

3. From mother to child

a. Before birth: virus crossing the placenta during pregnancy.

b. During birth: exposure to infected maternal blood and vaginal fluids.

c. After birth: ingesting breast milk containing the virus.

B. *Myths*. HIV is *not* transmitted through casual contact such as:

1. Drooling, biting, or contact with diapers in child care settings.

2. Daily contacts between family members, except through breastfeeding.

VI.   **Symptoms**. Pediatric HIV infection affects the immune system and also may act directly on specific organ systems. Children may not show symptoms at all or may show symptoms in many body systems.[11]

A.   Symptoms common in children under age 2 who have the HIV infection include

1.   fever,
2.   failure to thrive,
3.   weight loss,
4.   swollen or inflamed lymph nodes,
5.   enlarged liver or spleen,
6.   chronic diarrhea, and
7.   intractable oral thrush (an oral fungus infection that is not responsive to treatment).

B.   Damage to the central nervous system is also common, resulting in developmental delays and the loss of developmental milestones.

C.   Recurring bacterial infections are common because of damage to the immune system. Some infections now are more manageable with new medications.

D.   Other common symptoms include

1.   pulmonary (lung) abnormalities and different types of pneumonia;
2.   motor (movement) disturbances and muscle wasting;
3.   dermatitis (skin disorders);
4.   anemia and other blood disorders; and
5.   heart and kidney disorders.

---

[11]   "Diagnosis of Pediatric HIV Disease," by Y. A. Maldonado and A. Petru, in *The Aids Knowledge Book,* edited by P. T. Cohen, M. A. Sande, and P. A. Volberding (Boston: Little, Brown, 1994); and "Developmental Issues: Children Infected with the Human Immunodeficiency Virus," by C. B. Johnson, in *Infants and Young Children, 6*(1), 1-10.

VII. Treatments

A. Medications[12] may be prescribed to

1. prevent infections;

2. strengthen the immune system;

3. treat specific diseases, infections, and cancers; and

4. immunize against disease.

B. Nutritional support

C. Specialized therapies (physical, occupational, speech)

D. Treatments for pain

E. Special skin care

F. Early education intervention

G. Oxygen therapy[13]

VIII. Special care needs and interventions

A. A child with HIV is, first and foremost, a child who needs

1. comfort, hugs, and nurturing;

2. adequate and regular sleep;

---

[12] Administration of medication is generally regarded as an invasive procedure and, as such, is a nursing task that may be subject to statutory provisions or to regulations established by your State's Nursing Board. If this is the case, legislation or regulatory guidelines may be in place that determine whether or not and how this task may be delegated to a non-health-licensed individual (other than the child's parent or guardian). For the safety of the children, and due to the risk of personal and agency liability, you are urged to contact your State Board of Nursing to inquire about the status of delegation of invasive procedures in your state.

[13] Administration of oxygen therapy is an invasive procedure, and, therefore subject to state regulation in most states. You are urged to contact your State Board of Nursing so that policies and practices related to invasive procedures are in compliance with the law or related regulations or guidelines. These laws stipulate whether such procedures may or may not be performed by non-health licensed individuals, and the terms for delegation and supervision of these tasks.

3.　　proper nutrition;

4.　　opportunities for play and exploration;

5.　　opportunities for education and stimulation; and

6.　　opportunities to interact with others.

B.　Infection control

1.　Follow the special guidelines developed by the Centers for Disease Control and Prevention and the American Academy of Pediatrics (see Hotlines at the end of this module).

2.　Follow the general infection control guidelines for all children.

a.　Diapering

(1)　Keep diapering and cleaning supplies away from children.
(2)　Use a changing table made of plastic or formica, or table with a nonabsorbent pad.
(3)　Discard disposable diapers in a plastic-lined, covered container.
(4)　Store cloth diapers in plastic-lined, covered containers or individual plastic bags.
(5)　If using cloth diapers, launder them separately.
(6)　Store soiled clothing in individual plastic bags.
(7)　Place diapering area next to a handwashing sink.

b.　Handwashing

(1)　*Never* use handwashing sinks to prepare food, formula, or medication.[14]
(2)　Always help young children with handwashing after toileting, being diapered, blowing nose.
(3)　Use hand lotion after handwashing to prevent chapping.

---

[14] See footnote 12.

    c.   Gloves

        (1)   Use disposable gloves, *followed by handwashing*, when

            (a)   caregiver's hands have cuts or abrasions or are chapped;
            (b)   any child has diarrhea or a diagnosed infection;
            (c)   administering first aid to bloody wounds (keep disposable gloves in pockets on playground and on field trips); and
            (d)   handling bloody clothing, dressings, and so forth.

        (2)   *Do not* use the same pair of gloves with different children;
        (3)   *Do not* wash or attempt to disinfect gloves for additional use; and
        (4)   Dispose of gloves in plastic-lined, covered container.

    d.   Cleaning

        (1)   Use rubber gloves to prevent chapping.
        (2)   Use a bleach solution of 9 parts water to 1 part bleach that is made fresh daily.
        (3)   Use water at a temperature of 140°-160° F. for washing machines and dishwashers.
        (4)   Use water at a temperature of 110° F. or lower for children's handwashing sinks.
        (5)   Clean toys in dishwasher; wash separately from dishes and utensils.
        (6)   Dry laundry in a hot dryer.
        (7)   Clean and disinfect the telephone frequently.

3.   Avoiding contagious diseases

    a.   Follow correct handwashing and other infection control measures.
    b.   Be in compliance with proper immunizations (children and staff).

4.   Teach all children handwashing and other infection control and self-care techniques.

C.   Special care needs and interventions

    1.   Attitudes

        a.   Children with HIV and their families may be affected negatively by attitudes of others, including

           (1)   fear of rejection;
           (2)   prejudices about HIV infection and assumptions regarding family lifestyles;
           (3)   myths about how the virus is transmitted; and
           (4)   assumptions that the parent/guardian does not care for or love the child.

        b.   To deal with negative attitudes:

           (1)   Become educated with reliable materials that provide accurate information.
           (2)   Use materials for infection control (disposable gloves, bleach cleaning solutions, handwashing facilities) with all children. Wear gloves and masks only at appropriate times (such as when touching blood) and not in all cases when the child is touched.

    2.   Behavior

        a.   Children may demonstrate challenging or difficult behaviors if subject to

           (1)   an unstable home environment;
           (2)   effects of the illness or treatments;
           (3)   withdrawal from alcohol or other drugs;
           (4)   effects of alcohol or other drugs; or
           (5)   loss of family member.

        b.   Interventions to deal with challenging behaviors

           (1)   Provide quiet, friendly environments.
           (2)   Follow consistent and predictable routines.
           (3)   Help the child to develop and use appropriate coping skills.
           (4)   Control the amount of noise.
           (5)   Provide quiet time.

(6) Use music or rhythmic movements.
(7) Control the light level.
(8) Give consistent verbal and nonverbal messages.

3. Developmental issues

   a. Needs

     (1) Common problems include seizures, learning difficulties, and motor (movement) problems.
     (2) Children may have developmental lags as a result of the disease, lack of stimulation, or both.
     (3) Children may have been exposed to drugs during their mother's pregnancy and may have additional developmental complications.

   b. Interventions

     (1) Encourage and support the child's development, self-care skills, and independence.
     (2) Provide a safe, supportive environment, including any adaptations needed to ensure safety.

4. Expectations

   a. Parent/guardian, child, and caregivers must adapt continuously to ongoing changes caused by the infection.

     (1) The primary provider of care may change.
     (2) The parent or sibling(s) may have declining health or may die.
     (3) The child's health status may change, including more illness, over time.
     (4) Developmental delays, including loss of previously attained developmental milestones, may become more apparent.
     (5) The child's physical and emotional abilities may decline.
     (6) The child's need for intervention and treatment increases.

    b.   Interventions

        (1)   Consider the child with HIV as a child first.

        (2)   Provide the child with opportunities for play, exploration, and interaction.

        (3)   Provide consistent care that includes warmth, attention, and adequate nutrition.

        (4)   Incorporate specialized therapies and medications[15] as recommended and prescribed.

        (5)   Be sensitive to the family's task of coping with the child's changing health.

        (6)   Be aware that the child may be absent without notice because of changes in parental health status.

        (7)   Encourage the child's self-care skills, but adjust your expectations as the child's abilities decline.

5.   Parent and family issues

    a.   Needs

        (1)   Some parents have problems related to a wide range of factors.

            (a)   Parents who are HIV-infected are facing their own declining health and ultimate death from AIDS.

            (b)   Some parents have a substance abuse problem and may be unable to care for or be inconsistent in their care of the child.

            (c)   Many parents live in poverty and may not have access to resources including transportation.

            (d)   Parents are trying to deal with their own as well as their child's illness and eventual death.

        (2)   The people involved in a child's care may include extended family, friends, adoptive and foster parents.

---

[15] See footnote 12.

(a)   Families may be trying to cope with guilt, fear, and shame.

(b)   Families may be the target of discrimination and prejudice, which may block their access to and use of services and resources.

(c)   Families say isolation is their number-one problem.

(d)   Families may need referrals and information for medical care and financial assistance.

b.   Interventions

(1)   Be aware that the child, siblings, and parent(s) may be undergoing frequent medical procedures and hospitalizations.

(2)   Treat the child and family as normally as possible.

(3)   Maintain open communication with the family.

(4)   Show caring toward the child and family.

(5)   Be aware of community resources for families (such as substance abuse groups, HIV support groups, medical care, early intervention, hospices for counseling about death, dying, and bereavement issues).

6.   Legal issues

a.   Needs and concerns

(1)   Important laws that affect these children include Section 504 of the Rehabilitation Act, the Americans with Disabilities Act (ADA), and the Individuals with Disabilities Education Act (IDEA). They protect the rights of children with HIV to

(a)   participate in community settings with other children;

(b)   receive supportive services necessary for them to participate in community settings; and

(c)   participate without disclosure of HIV status unless the child's parents choose to disclose.

(2) These laws have implications for HIV testing, privacy/ confidentiality, range of services for which the children are eligible, and provision of a safe environment for children and employees.

b. Interventions

(1) Be aware of laws that affect children with HIV and their families.
(2) Follow policies instituted to meet legal requirements for caring for children with HIV and for maintaining a safe environment.
(3) Follow established guidelines regarding confidentiality of personal and medical information if a child's HIV-positive status is disclosed.
(4) Adhere to established policies that address public and parental concerns while preserving the rights of the child who has HIV infection.

7. Nutrition

a. Poor nutrition in children with HIV has many causes that may cause or contribute to

(1) anemia;
(2) failure to thrive;
(3) poor condition of the skin; and
(4) diarrhea.

b. Interventions to encourage better nutritional status

(1) Be patient during feedings and mealtimes.
(2) Provide a secure and consistent environment to ensure comfort during feeding.
(3) Allow the child extra rest to conserve energy for feeding.
(4) Give frequent meals, snacks, and fluids.
(5) Warm food and formula to lessen mouth pain.
(6) Enlarge nipple on bottle if necessary for easier feeding.

       (7)   Feed the child only special meals and formulas that are prescribed.

       (8)   Give any prescribed vitamins.[16]

       (9)   Cooperate with prescribed treatments, and monitor the child's response to treatments.

     (10)   Encourage adequate dental care.

     (11)   Be aware that breastfeeding is not recommended for mothers who have HIV-infection.

8.   Pain management

    a.   Needs

       (1)   Pain and discomfort are common.

       (2)   Skin and gastrointestinal problems affect the mouth, throat, stomach, and rectum.

    b.   Interventions

       (1)   Focus on reducing pain and increasing comfort.

       (2)   Attend to skin and gastrointestinal problems as directed by the child's health care provider.

       (3)   Administer any prescribed medications.[17]

       (4)   Use comfort strategies such as cuddling, quiet environment, soothing music, rocking, and carrying in snug sacks.

9.   Skin care

    a.   The child may have painful skin sores, infections, and rashes.

    b.   Interventions

       (1)   Follow established cleansing procedures.[18]

---

[16]   Physician-prescribed vitamins are a medication, the administration of which should be treated as an invasive procedure in accordance with state regulations.

[17]   See footnote 12.

[18]   See footnote 12.

    (2)   Give special attention to the skin during diapering and other skin cleansing.

    (3)   Give medication for pain as prescribed.[19]

    (4)   Be aware of nutritional principles to help improve skin condition.

BIBLIOGRAPHY

Betz, M. L. (1992). *Kindergartner with AIDS and the classroom barrier.* Horsham, PA: LRP Publications.

Crocker, A. C., Cohen, H. J., & Kastner, T. A. (Eds.) (1992). *HIV infection and developmental disabilities: A resource for service providers.* Baltimore: Paul H. Brooks.

Hausherr, R. (1989) *Children and the AIDS virus: A book for children, parents and teachers.* New York: Clarion Books.

Schilling, S., & Swain, J. (1990). *My name is Jonathan (and I have AIDS)* (teacher's edition). Denver: Prickly Pair Publishing & Consulting.

RESOURCES

AIDS Action Council, 1825 Connecticut Avenue NW, Suite 700, Washington, DC 20009; (202) 986-1300

Centers for Disease Control and Prevention (CDC), 1600 Clifton Road, Atlanta, GA 30333; (404) 639-3311

Child Welfare League of America, 440 First Street NW, Suite 310, Washington, DC 20001; (202) 638-2952

Healthy Mothers, Healthy Babies Coalition, 409-12th Street SW, Washington, DC 20024; (202) 863-2458

National AIDS Network, 729 Eighth Street SE, Suite 300, Washington, DC 20003; (202) 546-2424

Native American AIDS Prevention Center, 2100 Lake Shore Avenue, Suite A, Oakland, CA 94606; 1-800-283-AIDS ext. 2437

U. S. Public Health Service, Public Affairs Office Room 647-D, Hubert H. Humphrey Bldg., 200 Independence Avenue SW, Washington, DC 20201; (202) 690-7850

---

[19] See footnote 12.

Pediatric AIDS and HIV Infection: Fetus to Adolescent (Mhairi MacDonald and Harold Ginzberg, Eds.), Mary Ann Liebert Inc., 1651 Third Avenue, New York, NY 10128

Responding to HIV and AIDS, National Education Association Health Information Network, 1201-16th Street NW, Washington, DC 20036; (202) 822-7570

HOTLINES

CDC National AIDS Clearinghouse: 1-800-458-5231

National AIDS Hotline: 1-800-342-AIDS

National Institutes of Health (NIH): 1-800-243-7644

National Pediatric HIV Resource Center: 1-800-362-0071

Public Health Service AIDS hotlines

    1-800-344-7432 (Spanish)
    1-800-243-7889 (hearing impaired)
    1-800-283-7889 (American Indian)

EMOTIONAL PROBLEMS

I. **Common signs and symptoms of emotional problems**

    A.   Too little stimulation by parent or primary caregiver

    B.   Disturbed parent-child relationship

    C.   Underlying medical condition

    D.   Abuse or neglect

II. **Signs by age classification**

    A.   Newborn and young infant

        1.   A newborn or young infant normally will coo, laugh, and smile. In contrast, if the infant is listless and disinterested, or if the infant fails to thrive, an emotional problem may be present.

        2.   Infants born with physical problems such as blindness, deafness, skin disease, or prematurity may be listless and lethargic.

        3.   The infant may have serious problems with feeding, sleep, wakefulness, and may lack interest in or avoid adult attention.

    B.   Older infant (6-18 months)

        1.   Some behavior problems that may signal emotional problems are

            a.   excessive crying,
            b.   extreme anger and irritability,
            c.   refusal to eat, or
            d.   extreme apathy.

        2.   Stereotypic behaviors (constant repetition of certain meaningless gestures or movements) such as rocking, head rolling, staring at fingers, and other odd, repeated movements.

        3.   Failure to thrive

    4.   Abnormal attachment behaviors (such as unusual response or lack of response toward mother or failure to seek comfort from an adult when hurt or ill)

    5.   Not playing with toys normally

C.   Toddler

    1.   Developmental problems, especially in social and speech/language areas

    2.   Unusual timidity and fear of people

    3.   Problems with eating, sleeping, weaning, or toilet training

    4.   No interest in other children or troubled relationships with other children

    5.   Severe destructive behavior

    6.   Self-abusive behaviors

    7.   Stereotypic behaviors

    8.   Lack of flexible, constructive play

D.   Preschool-age child

    1.   Developmental problems, especially in social and speech/language areas

    2.   Problems with eating, sleeping, or toileting

    3.   No interest in other children, or troubled peer relations

    4.   Extreme shyness and withdrawal

    5.   Severe destructive behavior

    6.   Self-abusive behavior, suicidal threats

    7.   Stereotypic behaviors

    8.   Extreme hyperactivity

    9.   Aggression toward other children and adults

10. Temper tantrums that are extremely frequent or last for an extremely long time

11. Deliberate cruelty to animals

12. Fire setting

13. Lack of creative play, both pretend and with toys

14. Prolonged tearful, sad, low-energy moods, rapid and extreme changes in mood, severe or frequent episodes of defiance or hostility

15. Hoarding food or toys

16. Preoccupation with violence

17. Disorganized, disconnected thought patterns or speech patterns

18. Expression of emotions in an extreme and uncontrolled manner

III. Severe emotional disturbance

A. At all ages, severe emotional disturbance will be obvious to the caregiver. If you have questions about a child's behavior, speak with a supervisor or health or mental health professional.

B. Speak with parent/guardian immediately to explain your concerns. If professional help is available within your agency, get help immediately. If not, on a confidential basis (not identifying the child or family), seek advice from a health care professional on how to address issues with the family and how to be of assistance.

C. Children with severe emotional disturbances require professional health or mental health care.

D. Parent/guardian behavior toward and with the child

1. The child's parent/guardian may show signs of difficulty in relating to the child.

   a. Disappointment in child
   b. Dislike of child
   c. Impersonal toward child
   d. Extremely overanxious about child

e. Extremely overprotective of child
f. Depressed
g. Apathetic
h. Extremely hostile to child or to adults
i. Too rigid standards
j. Apprehension
k. Overreaction to normal child behaviors

2. History of abuse or neglect toward this or any other child.

IV. Caregiver actions

A. Observe and report.

1. Observe, record, and report to the parent/guardian any observed symptoms and suspicions of emotional problems.

2. Observe and record concerns about a child in a way that helps foster understanding of the child and is useful for communications with parents/guardians, health professionals, and mental health professionals.

B. Take the lead.

1. If interactions are uncomfortable, the caregiver can create a daily routine of interactions that is simple, playful, and mutually enjoyable.

2. Watch for the possibility of one worker or special caregiver (such as a foster grandparent) becoming a substitute mother in the child care setting.

C. Structure the setting.

1. Set extremely clear and consistent expectations and limits for toddlers and preschoolers.

2. Develop and follow a planned schedule of stimulation, socialization activities, play interactions, and consistent physical care.

D. Provide time and opportunities to practice new skills.

1. Use modeling and rehearsal.

2. Use guided and independent practice to increase the likelihood that the child will maintain new skills.

    E.   Build positive interactions with the child's family.

        1.   Over time, establish a daily habit of talking informally with the child's parent/guardian.

        2.   Without focusing on the problems too intensely at first, share information with the parent/guardian about the child's activities during the day.

        3.   Recognize that an informative, supportive, professional relationship may be the first step in helping a parent/guardian get professional help for the child.

    F.   Seek the assistance of medical or mental health professionals, if needed.

        1.   If the child seems to need additional professional services, schedule a conference with the parent/guardian, using observation notes to discuss concerns about the child.

        2.   Have available a list of two or three professional resources to give to the parent/guardian at this conference.

V.   Support services

    A.   Develop a resource list of professionals, organizations, and community agencies that serve children with emotional problems.

        1.   Use the list to help caregivers and parents/guardians locate specific services for a child with emotional problems.

        2.   Use the list to identify sources for additional caregiver training.

    B.   Resources in every community include

        1.   pediatricians and health care providers,

        2.   Child Find (through the local school district), and

        3.   local or county mental health clinics.

BIBLIOGRAPHY

Brazelton, T. B. (1994). *Touchpoints: Your child's emotional and behavioral development.* New York: Addison-Wesley.

Dwyer, K. P. (1990). Making the least restrictive environment work for children with serious emotional disturbance: Just say NO to segregated placements. *Preventing School Failure, 34*(3), 14-21.

Zeanah, C. H. (Ed.) (1993). *Handbook of infant mental health.* New York: Guilford Press.

RESOURCES

Autism Society of America, 7910 Woodmont Avenue, Suite 650, Bethesda, MD 20815; 1-800-328-8476

Autism Research Institute, 4182 Adams Avenue, San Diego, CA 92116; (619) 281-7165

CONGENITAL HEART DEFECTS

I. **Definition.** Incomplete or abnormal development of the heart in utero (while in the womb), resulting in deformities of the heart at birth.

II. **General categories of congenital heart defects**

    A. *Acyanotic* (pink) babies: skin coloring not affected and looks normal even though a heart defect is present.

    B. *Cyanotic* (blue) babies: unoxygenated or "blue" blood is circulated throughout the body, resulting in a bluish cast to the baby's skin.

III. **Signs and symptoms.** Vary depending on the type of heart defect. Many infants show no signs or symptoms.

    A. Congestive heart failure

        1. Extra blood flow to lungs places extra workload on the heart, causing it to pump less efficiently.

        2. Symptoms of the body's effort to compensate for the changes in heart and lung functioning include

            a. rapid breathing,
            b. rapid heart rate,
            c. tiring easily,
            d. sweating with feeding or even at rest or sleep,
            e. poor feeding (tires and is unable to take adequate quantities of formula),
            f. failure to thrive (poor weight gain), and
            g. frequent respiratory infections.

    B. Cyanotic heart defects

        1. Cyanosis (bluish cast to skin).

        2. Hypoxic spells: child becomes much bluer or grayish in color, very short of breath, and very limp, or possibly may pass out.

IV. **Pacemakers**

    A. A pacemaker is a surgically implanted device that maintains an adequate heart rate. Some (not most) children with pacemakers are totally dependent on these devices.

B.   A pacemaker may be called for because the child's heart beats irregularly or beats too rapidly or too slowly.

C.   Position of pacemaker in child may be

1.   just below left or right shoulder in front of chest,
2.   just below breastbone in upper portion of abdomen, or
3.   in abdomen.

D.   Most children with pacemakers have a telephone transmitter that allows pacemaker function to be checked by telephone. This is easy to do and does not hurt the child or cause any discomfort.

1.   Procedure

a.   Be sure that the child is sitting (or infant is lying) quietly.
b.   Slide wrist cuffs or finger cuffs over the hands or fingers.
c.   Turn on the unit.
d.   Having called the cardiologist or pacemaker clinic, now place handset of phone on transmitter for about 1 minute.

2.   A tracing of pacemaker activity will be transmitted to cardiologist or clinic for evaluation.

V.   **Special care needs**

A.   Asymptomatic children require no special interventions other than administration of medication (if prescribed).[1]

B.   Congestive heart failure

1.   Feeding

a.   Feed children slowly and often, as they breathe rapidly and tire easily.

---

[1]   Administration of medication is generally regarded as an invasive procedure and, as such, is a nursing task that may be subject to regulations established by your State's Nursing Board. If this is the case, legislation or regulatory guidelines may be in place that determine whether or not and how this task may be delegated to a non-health-licensed individual (other than the child's parent or guardian). For the safety of the children, and due to the risk of personal and agency liability, you are urged to contact your State Board of Nursing to inquire about the status of delegation of invasive procedures in your state.

        b.   Use formula (has more calories than juices) or solid food, or both, as directed.

        c.   If and as instructed, use concentrated formulas to increase calories per ounce.

  2.   Activity: Allow infants and children to set their own pace. Do not push them to do more than they feel like doing.

  3.   Medications[2]

        a.   Typical medications are:

           (1)   Lanoxin (Digoxin)

                (a)   strengthens heart muscle, and
                (b)   helps heart beat more effectively.

           (2)   Lasix (helps kidneys get rid of extra body fluid)

           (3)   Aldactone (Spirolactone)

                (a)   helps kidneys get rid of extra body fluid, and
                (b)   helps the body retain potassium, a mineral that helps the heart function normally.

        b.   These medications *must* be given on time and in the appropriate dose.

        c.   Parent/guardian should provide information about the child's medications, dosages, times, side effects, precautions, and a marked dropper or syringe for accurate administration.

        d.   A plan should be in place regarding what to do if the child vomits or spits up medication.

C.   Cyanotic heart defects

  1.   Activity: Allow these children to set their own pace.

---

[2] See footnote 1.

2. Hypoxic spell

    a. During the spell, place the child's knees on his/her chest, give oxygen as prescribed,[3] and call the physician.

    b. Observe

        (1) how the spell started (for example, crying, feeding, at rest),

        (2) duration,

        (3) the child's appearance during the spell, and

        (4) what the child was like after the spell.

D. Surgery

1. *Infection control:* Before and during the weeks following surgery, children with a heart defect may be more susceptible to infections. They should not be exposed to children with respiratory infections, runny nose, fever, strep infections, and the like.

2. *After surgery:*

    a. No hard blows to chest area; incision takes 6 weeks to heal.

    b. The child may need supplemental oxygen for a time.

    c. The child's wound should be healed over. Any areas that are still open must be kept clean, dry, covered, and inspected for any signs of infection.

        (1) Parent/guardian should provide any special instructions for care of wound.

        (2) During the first 2 weeks after surgery, parent/guardian should be contacted if the child has a fever.

3. *Activity:* Child should be allowed to set his/her limits.

---

[3] Administration of oxygen therapy is an invasive procedure and, therefore, subject to state regulation in most states. You are urged to contact your State Board of Nursing so that policies and practices related to invasive procedures are in compliance with the law or related regulations or guidelines. These laws stipulate whether such procedures may or may not be performed by non-health licensed individuals, and the terms for delegation and supervision of these tasks.

E. Children with pacemakers

1. *Information required* for children with pacemakers in child care setting

    a. Reason for pacemaker.
    b. Dependent on pacemaker or not?
    c. Location of the pacemaker on the child.
    d. Medications.
    e. Name and daytime phone number of parent/guardian.
    f. Name and phone number for emergency medical assistance.
    g. Telephone transmitter.
    h. Permission to contact the child's cardiologist or pacemaker clinic if pacemaker malfunctions or other emergency arises and the parent/guardian is unreachable.
    i. Acceptable activities; unacceptable activities.
    j. Lowest heart rate set for this child.

2. If the child has a *telephone transmitter:*

    a. Keep transmitter at child care center during the day while the child is there.
    b. List phone numbers including: parent/guardian (day numbers), cardiologist, pacemaker clinic, and nearest emergency facility.
    c. If the child with a pacemaker falls or injures himself/herself while at child care center, check pacemaker with telephone transmitter and contact parent/guardian.

3. If the child is totally *dependent on a pacemaker:*

    a. Have readily available the emergency plan in written form.
    b. Have prior training in cardiopulmonary respiration (CPR).

4. *Pacemaker malfunction*

    a. If the pacemaker stops or malfunctions, the child

        (1) may pass out;
        (2) may complain of dizziness, light-headedness, or headaches; or

(3)   may tire easily or fall asleep easily, sleep longer, and sleep more often. Infants may fall asleep during feeding or have no energy to feed at all.

b.   A child who is totally dependent on a pacemaker requires immediate emergency CPR intervention to survive. This is a medical emergency for which CPR should be started as soon as the child has no heart rate, or sooner if specified in the emergency plan.

5.   *Special considerations* for children with pacemakers

a.   The child must avoid the following:

(1)   Magnets and strong radiowaves (present inside a radio station or in the vicinity of a "ham" radio. (The following do *not* pose a threat: CB radios, electronic appliances, microwave ovens.)

(2)   Trampolines and jumping from heights (such as out of trees, off fences, off desks) (although jumping jacks and active play are permitted).

(3)   Contact sports (such as contact football) or any sport in which the child might receive a hard blow to the chest or abdomen.

b.   The child may take part in activities such as crawling, running, swimming, and general playground activities.

F.   *General considerations* for children with congenital heart disease and pacemakers

1.   *Encouragement.* Each child should be encouraged to reach his/her maximum potential. This does not mean "pushing" the child to achieve but, instead, stimulating and encouraging him/her to do as much as possible.

a.   Emphasis should be on what the child *can* do, not what he/she cannot do. Instead of saying, "You can't do this," say, "Why don't you do this instead?" Then help the child to become interested in the alternative activity.

b.   Children need to feel good about themselves and their abilities and need praise for accomplishments, even small ones.
c.   Children who receive caring interactions specific to their needs in a positive environment are more likely to develop a healthy self-image than to become angry and fixated on their limitations.

2.   *Activity parameters* for children with congenital heart disease and pacemakers. (Individual specific limitations have been discussed already under the various types of heart conditions.)

a.   Infants need stimulation with mobiles and bright colors, and to be talked to, held, sung to, to look in mirrors, and the like.
b.   Older infants need to flex their muscles, kick, crawl, play in water, use safe toys, be sung and talked to, and so on.
c.   Older children need active play, such as running and swimming. If these activities are not possible, the child can be stimulated through more sedentary tasks such as fingerpainting and cutouts.

BIBLIOGRAPHY

American Heart Association (1981). *If your child has a congenital heart defect: A guide for parents.* Dallas: AHA.

Jackson, P. L., & Vessey, J. (1992). *Primary care of the child with a chronic condition.* St. Louis: Mosby.

Moller, J., & Neal, W. (Eds.) (1990). *Fetal, neonatal and infant cardiac disease.* Norwalk, CT: Appleton & Lange.

RESOURCES

American Heart Association: 1-800-242-8721

MAJOR RESPIRATORY DISEASES IN CHILDHOOD

I.   Asthma

A.   Asthma is a chronic lung disease with the following characteristics:

    1.   Swelling of the lining of airways

    2.   Temporary blocking or narrowing of the airways causing less air flow

    3.   More sensitivity of the airway triggers (discussed under E.) that cause more mucus, which plugs airways.

B.   Frequency

    1.   Prevalence of asthma in the general population is 13,074,000, of which 4,830,000 cases are in children under age 18.[1]

    2.   Incidence of asthma is highest in childhood; first attack usually occurs before age 5. Asthma often disappears with time.

    3.   Boys are more likely than girls to have asthma until age 10, then both equally.

    4.   Asthma tends to run in families, but other factors, such as past viral respiratory illnesses, also play a role.

C.   Special problems in early childhood

    1.   Infants, toddlers, and young children have smaller airways than older children, and these airways can become blocked quite easily.

    2.   Young children catch colds and other infections more easily than older children because their immune systems are not fully developed. This creates more frequent problems for children with asthma.

---

[1] Source: National Institute of Health, Atlanta, 1993 data.

D. Course of the illness

    1.   Symptoms may disappear as the child reaches school age or adolescence, but predicting who and when is difficult. Some experts believe that the fewer attacks a child has, the better the long term outlook is.

    2.   Well controlled asthma should result in times when the child has no symptoms.

E. Triggers

    1.   Definition and important points

        a.   Triggers are things that make asthma symptoms appear or worsen.

        b.   A child may have one or many triggers, which may change over time.

        c.   Triggers should be avoided when possible. Or the physician may recommend pretreatment with an inhaled medication before a child is exposed to triggers that can't be avoided, such as exercise.

    2.   Types of triggers

        a.   Irritants including

            (1)   smoke (from cigarette, pipe, cigar, fireplace);

            (2)   strong odors (perfume, paint fumes, cleaning solutions);

            (3)   dust (indoors or outdoors);

            (4)   air pollution; and

            (5)   aerosol sprays.

        b.   Allergens (things that may cause reactions in allergic children) including

            (1)   environmental triggers such as

                (a)   animal dander from furry or feathered creatures (cat and rabbit are most common);

                (b)   dust mites (microscopic animals that live in dust, especially in mattresses and overstuffed furniture); and

          (c)   indoor and outdoor molds, pollens from plants (particularly weeds).

    (2)   foods such as

          (a)   dairy products,
          (b)   nuts, and
          (c)   shellfish.

    (3)   medications such as

          (a)   aspirin, and
          (b)   antibiotics.

  c.   Infections including

    (1)   common cold viruses,
    (2)   sinusitis (infection of the sinuses), and
    (3)   influenza.

  d.   Weather including

    (1)   quick change in weather or barometric pressure, and
    (2)   wind.

  e.   Vigorous exercise
  f.   Strong emotions such as

    (1)   laughing or crying (increased air flow and jerky breathing pattern may trigger asthma),
    (2)   anger, and
    (3)   stress.

F.   Monitoring

  1.   Peak flow meter: an instrument used to measure air flow in children 4 years and older.

    a.   *Operation.* The child blows as hard as he or she can into the peak flow meter, which moves an arrow up to a number on the meter. (A good effort is needed for reliable readings.)
    b.   *Interpretation.* The goal number is specific for each child but will be higher if air flow is not blocked and lower if it is blocked.

   2.   Early warning signs (EWS) of asthma are things that happen *before* the start of an asthma episode. Each child will have his/her own EWS, which may change over time.

        a.   Young children may not be aware of these signs. Therefore, caregivers must be aware of each child's specific signs and be alert to their onset so early treatment steps can begin. Early treatment will help prevent more severe symptoms.

        b.   EWS include the following:[2]

Breathing slows down	Looks pale
Eyes look glassy	Acts tired
Gets upset easily	Wants to be alone
Acts sad, mopey	Acts quiet
Acts excited	Has dark circles
Acts nervous, restless	under eyes
Eyes water	Acts grumpy
Feels clammy	Has runny nose
Feels feverish	Sneezes
Complains of scratchy	Coughs
or itchy throat	

G.   Symptoms. These are unique to each child, but typical symptoms include the following:

   1.   Wheezing, a high-pitched sound heard when the child breathes (may not be heard without a stethoscope)

   2.   Cough (many young children cough instead of wheeze)

   3.   Shortness of breath

   4.   Complaints of tightness or pain in chest

   5.   Increased respiratory and heart rate

   6.   Peak flow numbers significantly lower than typical (more than 20% drop)

---

[2] Adapted from a video, *Learning About Asthma,* by permission of National Jewish Center for Immunology and Respiratory Medicine, Denver, CO.

H.   Severe asthma symptoms with respiratory distress.

1.   Unusual posture (hunched shoulders)

2.   Nasal flaring (nostrils get bigger when child breathes in)

3.   Breathing through the mouth

4.   Retractions (skin between ribs and above and below breastbone pulls inward with breathing)

5.   Difficulty talking or breathlessness

6.   Changes in skin color — blue or gray around mouth, fingernails (VERY SERIOUS SIGN!)

7.   Peak flow numbers very low; child may be unable to blow at all (more than 40% drop)

I.   Special care needs of children with asthma

1.   General guidelines

a.   Learn each child's triggers and avoid exposing the child to them if possible.

b.   Follow good handwashing to reduce the risk of infection.

c.   Be aware that influenza vaccine may reduce the frequency of infections.

d.   Give medications as prescribed by physician and caregivers.[3] Administer prescribed preventive treatment 10-15 minutes before exercise to help prevent asthma symptoms during or after exercise.

e.   To reduce episodes triggered by weather:

(1)   Be sure the child's asthma is under control;

---

[3]   Administration of medication is generally regarded as an invasive procedure and, as such, is a nursing task that may be subject to regulations established by your State's Nursing Board. If this is the case, legislation or regulatory guidelines may be in place that determines whether or not and how this task may be delegated to a non-health-licensed individual (other than the child's parent or guardian). For the safety of the children, and due to the risk or personal and agency liability, you are urged to contact your State Board of Nursing to inquire about the status of delegation of invasive procedures in your state.

(2)   Minimize the child's exposure to wind and cold air (for example, wrap a scarf around the nose and mouth;

(3)   Administer medications exactly on time.

f.   Have available a clearly spelled-out plan for mild, moderate, and severe symptoms, including an emergency action plan.

g.   Discipline the child the same as other children. Do not overprotect the child.

h.   Involve the child in the same play activities as other children if health permits. Asthmatic children should remain as active as possible so they will have fun, stay fit, and develop normally.

i.   Instill regular daily routines.

2.   See Table 1 for a summary of what to do when warning signals arise.

Table 1
What to Do for Asthma[4]

Symptoms	What to Do
Early Warning Signs	
Cough Mild wheezing Hunched shoulders	Have child relax and use abdominal breathing
More Serious Signs	
Wheezing or trouble breathing out Decreased breath sounds or shallow breathing Increased heart rate Cough	Check pulse rate Call parent/guardian
Very Serious Signs	
Retractions (pulling in of spaces below or between ribs or above collarbone) Nasal flaring Blueness of nail beds Severe decrease in breath sounds	Call emergency help Call parent/guardian

---

[4]   Source: Adapted from a handout, *What to Do for Asthma,* by permission from the National Jewish Center for Immunology and Respiratory Medicine, Denver, CO.

3.   Medications

   a.   Bronchodilator (for example, Albuterol, Proventil)

   (1)   relaxes muscles around airways (Albuterol is fast-acting when inhaled); and
   (2)   can be taken by inhalation, syrup, or capsules.

   b.   Anti-inflammatory drugs (Cromolyn, Prednisone, and other)

   (1)   reduce swelling inside the airways (slow-acting); and
   (2)   can be taken be inhalation, syrup, or tablets.

4.   Relaxation, through stories, music, or being held (may be used along with medications)

II.   Bronchopulmonary dysplasia (BPD)

A.   Bronchopulmonary dysplsia (BPD) is a condition of premature infants in which sensitive, generally immature lungs become inflamed.

B.   Many children will experience developmental delays for the first 24-36 months of life. This is related directly to the length, number, and intensity of the hospitalizations and, therefore, lack of stimulation the child experienced in early life. Every system, such as musculoskeletal, gastrointestinal, cardiac, and central nervous system, may be affected.

C.   Nutrition and hydration: May need to eat and drink small amounts frequently

D.   Environmental control: Eliminate all forms of smoke and allergy-producing items

E.   Therapy

1.   Oxygen

2   May require routine inhalant therapies: bronchial dilators and anti-inflammatory medications

        3.   Chest percussion
        4.   Oral medications

   F.   Outcome determined by state of health following hospital discharge and not solely by initial injury to the lungs.

        1.   Slow, steady improvement

        2.   Some toddlers have a mild intolerance to exercise as a residual effect.

III. Cystic fibrosis (CF)

   A.   Cystic fibrosis is a genetic disease affecting the exocrine (mucous-producing) glands in which secretions of thick mucus prevent normal functioning of body organs (most commonly, lungs, digestive system, and sweat glands).

   B.   Incidence[5]

        1.   Most common lethal inherited disease affecting Caucasian children in the U.S. (1 in 2,000 - 2,500 births).

        2.   Less frequent in African-Americans (1 in 17,000 births).

        3.   Asians and American Indians rarely affected.

   C.   Course

        1.   Affected individuals are surviving longer.

        2.   Delays in physical growth are common, but development of intelligence and thinking skills are unaffected.

   D.   Common problems

        1.   Chronic or recurring infections of the respiratory tract

        2.   Difficulty digesting food (and failure to thrive) because of needed enzymes from pancreas

        3.   Chronic cough (not contagious)

---

[5] Source: Cystic Fibrosis Foundation, Patient Registry Data Report, August 1994, Bethesda, MD

      4.   Stools that may be more frequent than in typical children, foul smelling, and accompanied by cramping and gas related to poor digestion of fats.

E.   Special care needs of children with cystic fibrosis

    1.   General guidelines

        a.   Be consistent in behavioral expectations and discipline.
        b.   Report stooling patterns to the parent/guardian regularly or when changes occur.
        c.   Point out anything that is missing in the child's immunizations and annual flu shots.
        d.   Allow the child adequate rest, but encourage exercise to help general health, heart/lung condition, and developmental progress.
        e.   Be sure the family is aware of the Cystic Fibrosis Foundation as a resource.

    2.   Intervention

        a.   Chest physical therapy (CPT), clapping on (or vibrating) the child's chest in different positions to promote drainage as recommended by the health care professional and family

        b.   Medications include

            (1)   inhaled bronchodilator medication (given before chest physical therapy),
            (2)   antibiotics, and
            (3)   anti-inflammatory drugs.

    3.   Nutrition and hydration

        a.   Oral pancreatic enzyme replacement as prescribed[6]
        b.   More calories in diet
        c.   More protein in diet
        d.   More salt in diet
        e.   More fluids

---

[6] See footnote 3.

BIBLIOGRAPHY

Bancalari, E., & Stocker, J. T. (Eds.) (1988). *Bronchopulmonary dysplasia.* Hemisphere Publishing.

Celano, M. P., & Geller, R. J. (1993). Learning, school performance, and children with asthma: How much at risk? *Journal of Learning Disabilities, 26*(1), 23-32.

Cunningham, J. C., & Taussig, L. (1995). *An introduction to cystic fibrosis.* Bethesda, MD: Cystic Fibrosis Foundation.

Hogshead, N. & Couzens, G. (1990). *Asthma and exercise.* New York: Holt.

Jackson, D. F. (1986). Nursing care plan: Home management of children with BPD. *Pediatric Nursing, 10,* 342-348.

Jackson, P. L., and Vessey, J. A. (1992). *Primary care of the child with a chronic condition.* St. Louis: Mosby Year Book.

McMullen, A. H. (1992): Cystic fibrosis. In P. L. Jackson & J. A. Vessey (Eds.), *Primary care the child with a chronic condition* (pp. 210-228). St. Louis: Mosby Year Book.

Mrazek, D. A. (1993). Psychosomatic processes and physical illnesses. In C. H. Zeanah (Ed.), *Handbook of infant mental health* (pp. 350-358). New York: Guilford Press.

Mullen, A. & Oliver, S. (1994). *The asthma wizzard activity book.* Denver: National Jewish Center for Immunology and Respiratory Medicine.

Newhouse, M. T., & Barnes, P. J. (1991). *Conquering asthma: An illustrated guide to understanding and care for adults and children.* Toronto: Decker Periodicals.

Plaut, T. (1990). *One-minute asthma.* Amherst, MA: Pedipress Inc.

Sander, N. (1989). *A parent's guide to asthma.* New York: Doubleday.

Shayevitz, M. B., & Shayevitz, B. R. (1991). *Living well with chronic asthma, bronchitis, and emphysema.* Yonkers, NY: Consumer Reports Books.

Weinstein, A. (1990). *Asthma: The complete guide to self-management of asthma and allergies for patients and their families.* New York: McGraw-Hill.

RESOURCES

American Academy of Allergy and Immunology, 611 East Wells St., Milwaukee, WI 53202; 1-800-822-2762; (414) 272-6071

Asthma and Allergy Foundation of America, (educational materials, newsletter, videos family support groups), 1717 Massachusetts Avenue, Washington, DC 20036; 1-800-7-ASTHMA or (202) 466-7643

Cystic Fibrosis Foundation, 6931 Arlington Road, Bethesda, MD 20814; 1-800-FIGHT-CF

National Jewish Center for Immunology and Respiratory Medicine, 1400 Jackson Street, Denver, CO 80206; 1-800-222-LUNG

Booklets available from the National Jewish Center for Immunology and Respiratory Medicine:

- *Learning About Asthma: An Asthma Education Program* (1989)
- *Management of Chronic Respiratory Disease* (1987)
- *Your Child and Asthma* (1992)

Videos available from the National Jewish Center for Immunology and Respiratory Medicine:

- *A Breath Away* (1994)
- *Learning About Asthma* (1994)
- *Monitoring Your Asthma with a Peak Flow Meter* (1994)

For additional information and a monthly newsletter:

Mothers of Asthmatics, Inc., 3554 Chain Bridge Road, Fairfax, VA 22030; 1-800-878-4403 or (703) 385-4403

Asthma and Allergy Foundation of America, 1717 Massachusetts Avenue, Washington, DC 20036,1-800-7-ASTHMA
(educational materials, newsletter, videos, family support groups)

APNEA MONITORING

I. Defining and characterizing apnea

A. Apnea is a condition characterized by cessation of breathing for 20 seconds or longer, or shorter episodes associated with *bradycardia* (heart rate below 80 in an infant), *cyanosis* (color change in which lips, nailbeds, or skin around eyes may have a bluish hue), or *pallor* (paleness).

B. Differences between apnea and periodic breathing

1. Periodic breathing occurs when the infant stops breathing for 5 - 10 seconds, then starts breathing spontaneously again.

2. All infants have brief pauses in breathing and slight breathing irregularities.

3. Unlike apnea, periodic breathing is considered normal in an infant.

4. Periodic breathing frequently occurs when an infant is sleeping.

C. Differences between apnea and near SIDS (Sudden Infant Death Syndrome)

1. There is no such thing as "near SIDS."

2. Apnea has specific causes and potential risk factors, whereas the cause or causes of SIDS are not yet known.

II. Potential causes and risk factors associated with apnea

A. Infants, toddlers, and young children with disorders of the nervous system (seizure disorders)

B. Premature infants with immature nervous system

C. Infants of mothers who abused cocaine or opiates

D. Infants with congenital facial or airway defects

E. Infants with hypotonia (floppy muscles) who are not positioned correctly

F.   Infants with gastroesophageal reflux (regurgitation of stomach contents into the esophagus), which may result in difficulty coordinating swallowing and breathing; most common during feeding and burping.

G.   Infants, toddlers, and young children with a variety of respiratory or cardiac problems

H.   Infants, toddlers, and young children with tracheostomies (if the tube becomes blocked)

III.   What to do when infant is not breathing

A.   Observe the infant.

1.   Without disturbing the baby, check skin color and look to see if he/she is breathing.

2.   To check for breathing, watch for chest movement and put your ear near the infant's mouth and nose and listen for breathing.

3.   If the infant is

a.   not breathing but skin color is normal, wait 10 seconds to see if he/she will start breathing again spontaneously;
b.   cyanotic (bluish skin color, especially around the mouth and nailbeds) *or* does not start breathing within 10 seconds, follow these four steps:

(1)   Lay the infant on his/her back;
(2)   Stimulate the infant first by touching him/her;
(3)   Gently shake the infant; and
(4)   Slap the bottoms of the infant's feet.

4.   If these measures do not work, call for help and start CPR.

IV.   Home monitors

A.   A monitor is a mechanical device that detects breathing or heart rate, or both.

B. Types of monitors

　　1.　Apnea monitor: used only to document stoppages of breathing in infants.

　　2.　Combination apnea and bradycardia (slow heartbeat) monitor: sounds an alarm if infant stops breathing or heart rate drops below a set rate.

　　3.　Mattress monitor: measures simple chest wall movements.

　　4.　Impedance monitor: measures heart rate and respiratory effort (breathing); applied to infant either with sticky electrodes or with a belt placed across the chest.

C. Functions of a monitor

　　1.　The monitor provides 24-hour surveillance of the infant's breathing or breathing plus heart rate (to do this, it must be hooked up correctly and alarm limits set accurately).

　　2.　The monitor alarm will sound when it senses that breathing (or heart rate) has dropped below a preset level.

　　3.　A monitor is *not* a cure for apnea. It is only a device that will alert caregivers that the infant may need assistance.

D. Who needs a monitor?

　　1.　Infants who have had a documented apneic event that required CPR or vigorous stimulation

　　2.　Infants who are at high risk to have an apneic event (discussed under II)

E. Use of monitor

　　1.　A health care professional who knows the child well should instruct the caregiver on how to operate the child's monitor.

2. Operating information includes

    a. how the limits for the alarms (respiratory and cardiac) are set and how to check them in case the settings are changed accidentally;

    b. how to connect leads to the child and to the monitor properly;

    c. if monitor has a back-up battery, how to change batteries (make sure parent/guardian supplies an extra set of batteries;

    d. who to contact if equipment breaks (malfunctions); and

    e. user's guide or instruction manual provided by the monitor manufacturer.

F. What to do when the monitor sounds an alarm

1. Respond immediately.

2. Look at the monitor quickly to see why it is going off. Monitors have audio or visual alarms, or both, to tell you if the infant's heart rate or breathing rate is too low, or both.

3. Focus your attention on the *child,* not on the monitor. Check to see if child is blue, and whether he/she is breathing.

4. Follow steps already discussed (under III) on what to do if the infant is not breathing.

5. Record

    a. the infant's color, heart rate, and breathing rate;
    b. how long the episode lasted;
    c. your intervention; and
    d. the infant's response to your intervention.

G. Conditions that may cause false alarms of monitor

1. Loose monitor leads

2. Improper placement of lead or belt

3. Infant movement that pulls leads off

4. Dry or cracked electrodes

5.   Incorrect sensitivity adjustment

6.   Monitor wires hooked up incorrectly

H.   Safety guidelines for using monitors

1.   Placement and operation

a.   Place monitor on a solid, flat surface.
b.   Make sure monitor is several feet away from electrical devices such as air conditioner, TV, remote telephones.
c.   Do not use extension cords (some put out interference that can affect accurate functioning of the equipment).
d.   Unplug power cord from the wall if it is unplugged from the monitor.
e.   Have battery pack or electrical system available.

2.   Response to alarms

a.   Make sure monitor alarm is on and audible wherever you are.
b.   Respond immediately to any monitor alarm.
c.   If necessary, perform CPR according to your certified training.

3.   Child safety

a.   Supervise the child closely to make sure he/she does not disconnect the monitor.
b.   Before bathing an infant, remove monitor electrodes and turn off the monitor.
c.   Remove leads from infants when they are not attached to the monitor.

V.   Special needs of children on monitors

A.   Emotional

1.   Treat children with apnea like all other children. All children need to be held, cuddled, and stimulated.

2.   Unhook children from their monitors when they are awake, as long as an adult is observing them. Check with the child's health care professional and parent/guardian regarding that specific child's monitoring.

B. Skin care

1. Remove electrodes from the skin at least every 3 days (or more often if they are loose), and wash and dry the skin under the electrodes.

2. Observe the skin for any signs of irritation (redness or rash).

3. When replacing electrodes, do not place over the child's nipples.

4. Do not use lotions where electrodes are placed (this can cause false alarms or make it difficult to attach electrodes.)

BIBLIOGRAPHY

Ahmann, E., Meany, R. G., & Fink, R. J. (1992). Use of home apnea monitors. *Journal of Obstetric, Gynecologic, & Neonatal Nursing, 21*(5), 394-399.

Keens, T. G., & Davidson Ward, S. L. (1993). Apnea spells, sudden death, and the role of the apnea monitor. *Pediatric Clinics of North America, 40*(5), 897-911.

Whitaker, S. (1995). The art and science of home infant apnea monitoring in the 1990s. *Journal of Obstetric, Gynecologic, & Neonatal Nursing, 24*(1), 84-89.

CHILDREN WITH SEIZURES

I.   **Definitions**

    A.   *Seizure:* a sudden, unusual discharge of electrical energy in the brain.

        1.   The discharge of energy may involve most of the brain (a generalized seizure) or just part of the brain (a partial or focal seizure).

        2.   The part of the body affected by the seizure is determined by the part or parts of the brain affected.

        3.   A seizure results from abnormal brain function, either temporary or long-lasting.

    B.   *Epilepsy:* a chronic condition characterized by repeated, unprovoked seizures.

    C.   *Status epilepticus:* a prolonged seizure, or series of uncontrolled seizures that continue without stopping, usually 20 minutes or more; a medical emergency.

II.   **Incidence**[1]

    A.   About 1,000 in 100,000 people in the United States will seek medical attention for a newly recognized seizure.

    B.   Epilepsy is the most common neurologic (affecting the nerves) problem in children.

    C.   Infants are more likely than any other age group to have seizures.

    D.   The rate of epilepsy in preschool children is about 1 in 50.

III.   **General characteristics**

    A.   Close to half of children who have seizures will improve as they get older.

    B.   Between seizures most people are able to function normally and are healthy.

---

[1]   Source: Epilepsy Foundation of America

IV.   **Causes of seizures in young children**

    A.   Epilepsy has no single cause; it can result from any number of conditions that injure the brain or affect its function.

    B.   Seizures may be caused by

        1.   familial or genetic factors,

        2.   abnormalities of the chromosomes, such as Down syndrome,

        3.   injury to the child's brain when in the womb or during delivery,

        4.   poisoning,

        5.   prematurity or critical illness in the first month of life,

        6.   childhood infections,

        7.   head injury of any type,

        8.   progressive brain disease, and/or

        9.   fever.

V.   **Treatment of seizures**

    A.   Most epilepsy can be treated, allowing the affected person to lead a normal life.

    B.   About half of people with seizures can expect full control of their seizures.

    C.   Drug therapy is the most common form of treatment.

    D.   A special diet is effective to control seizures in a small number of people.

    E.   If medications fail to control the seizures, brain surgery may be done in the most severe cases.

    F.   About 75% of people with seizures can be treated in their local community.

VI. **Effect of epilepsy on the child and family**

    A.   Negative public attitudes toward people with epilepsy may be a bigger problem than the condition itself.

    B.   Parents/guardians tend to overprotect the child with epilepsy.

    C.   Children with seizures have higher risk for developmental delays and slower emotional maturity.

    D.   Children with seizures have higher risk for problems with learning and attention.

    E.   Infants with frequent seizures may have difficulty eating and may not gain enough weight.

    F.   Children with epilepsy have a greater risk of developing emotional/behavioral problems, including low self-esteem.

    G.   Families with a child with epilepsy undergo increased stress.

VII. **General characteristics of a seizure**

    A.   *Aura:* a sensation such as a smell, memory, feeling, or sound that occurs just before a seizure.

    B.   *Prodrome:* a feeling of fear or anxiety that occurs days or hours before a seizure.

    C.   *Eye movement:* eyes may roll back or move to one side or the other, or move jerkily.

    D.   *Muscle movement:* a regular, rhythmic pattern of muscle movement in the area of the body affected.

    E.   Impairment or *loss of consciousness* or unresponsiveness.

    F.   *Pallor* of face or bluish color around lips and/or nailbeds.

    G.   *Post-ictal state:* a period of time after a seizure when the child is sleepy, lethargic, or not himself/herself.

VIII. **Types of seizures**

    A.   Generalized tonic-clonic (grand mal)

        1.   May occur at any age.

2. Symptoms include loss of consciousness, stiffening and shaking of entire body.

3. Child may be pale or have a bluish color around the mouth.

4. Usually lasts 2-5 minutes; may last up to 15 minutes.

5. Followed by a post-ictal state.

B. Absence seizures (petit mal)

1. More common in children age 5-15 years and rare in children younger than 3 years.

2. Most common type of seizure disorder.

3. Characterized by a "staring spell."

4. Usually last less than 15 seconds.

6. May occur frequently (100 times a day).

7. Child may not realize the seizure has occurred.

C. Atonic seizures (drop attacks)

1. May occur in infants through school-age children.

2. Child suddenly collapses and falls; an infant may slump over.

3. Child recovers in 10 seconds to 1 minute, regains consciousness.

4. Child may be injured in falling.

D. Myoclonic seizures

1. May occur in infants through adolescents.

2. Usually associated with other neurologic problems and developmental delays.

3. Occur as sudden, brief muscle jerks that involve all or part of the body.

4. Child may drop things or fall.

5.   Child may be injured in falling.

E.   Simple partial seizures

1.   Child may see or feel unusual sensations.

2.   May turn pale, sweat, or flush.

3.   May complain of feeling sick.

4.   One part of the body may jerk, progressing throughout the body.

5.   Unusual in young children.

F.   Complex partial seizures

1.   Rare in infants and toddlers.

2.   Child may appear confused, clumsy, may wander off.

3.   Usually last a few minutes.

4.   Child may have post-ictal confusion.

5.   Safety precautions are necessary.

G.   Infantile spasms

1.   A syndrome of symptoms that includes seizures.

2.   Occur in infants 3-12 months of age.

3.   May appear as a nod of the head or a total body jerk, a "jackknife" movement.

4.   Tend to occur in clusters.

5.   Associated with developmental delays.

H.   Febrile seizures

1.   Occur during a fever.

2.   Characterized by generalized, convulsive-type movements of the body.

3.   Most occur between 6 and 36 months of age.

I.   Common conditions that include seizures

   1.   Lenox-Gastaut syndrome

      a.   Starts in early childhood, ages 1-5 years.
      b.   Includes various types of seizures.
      c.   Associated with mental retardation and developmental delay

   2.   Benign focal epilepsy

      a.   Starts around 4-10 years of age.
      b.   Seizures occur during sleep.
      c.   Seizure starts with twitching of the face, then spreads to other parts of the body.
      d.   Usually disappears during adolescence.

   3.   Cerebral palsy: About one-third of children with cerebral palsy have seizures.

IX.   **Seizure-like conditions**

   A.   Breath-holding

      1.   Happens because of fright, frustration, or anger.

      2.   Is not a seizure, but parent/guardian should be notified.

   B.   Gastroesophogeal reflux

      1.   A condition in infants that produces frequent vomiting.

      2.   Looks like a "convulsion," but is not a seizure.

      3.   Child is at risk of choking.

      4.   Child should be evaluated by a physician.

   C.   Migraines

      1.   Headache may or may not be present.

      2.   Other symptoms are vomiting, nausea, diarrhea, flushing or pallor, intolerance to light, and/or confusion.

3. Requires evaluation by a physician but is not an emergency.

X. Medications to control seizures

A. General considerations

1. Most children's seizures can be controlled by medication.

2. Children might take one or more kinds of seizure medication.

3. Seizure medications may make children sleepy or alter their ability to pay attention.

4. Some medications have undesirable side effects.

5. The child should be observed for side effects of the medication and, if any, the parent/guardian informed.

B. Types of medications[2]

1. The most commonly prescribed antiepileptic medications are:

    a. Dilantin (phenytoin)
    b. Depakene/Depakote (valproic acid/divalproex sodium)
    c. Tegretol (carbamazepine)
    d. Phenobarbital
    e. Felbatol (felbamate) is a new medication (as of 1993) that may take the place of Depakene/Depakote

---

[2] Administration of medication is generally regarded as an invasive procedure and, as such, is a nursing task that may be subject to statutory provisions or to regulations established by your State's Nursing Board. If this is the case, legislation or regulatory guidelines may be in place that determine whether or not and how this task may be delegated to a non-health-licensed individual (other than the child's parent or guardian). For the safety of the children, and due to the risk of personal and agency liability, you are urged to contact your State Board of Nursing to inquire about the status of delegation of invasive procedures in your state.

XI.   **Safety considerations.** Factors that may increase the risk of seizures in a child with a known seizure disorder include

    A.   stress,

    B.   increasing or decreasing doses of medication,

    C.   illness,

    D.   inadequate sleep,

    E.   periods of rapid growth, and

    F.   blinking or flashing lights.

XII.   **Care of the child during a seizure**

    A.   When you first observe signs of a seizure

        1.   turn the child to side (or child's head to the side);

        2.   try to clean out the mouth and nose to prevent choking if child has vomited;

        3.   do not try to force the child's mouth open or put anything in his/her mouth;

        4.   remove hard objects from thrashing range, but do not restrain;

        5.   place a blanket or pillow under the child's head;

        6.   remove tight, restrictive clothing;

        7.   stay with the child throughout the seizure;

        8.   do not try to give the child food, drink, or a bottle until he/she is fully awake; and

        9.   time the episode with a watch.

    B.   An emergency situation exists if

        1.   the seizure lasts more than 20 minutes, OR

        2.   the child has continuous seizures, OR

    3.   the child remains unconscious after the seizure, OR

    4.   he/she stops breathing.

  C.   Contact emergency medical assistance, start CPR if appropriate, and contact the child's parent/guardian.

XIII. **Observation and recording of the seizure** (important to give parent/guardian and the child's physician an accurate description of the seizure)

XIV. **The child with a known seizure disorder**

  A.   Discuss with the child's parent/guardian the plan for care if the child has a seizure.

  B.   Ask the parent/guardian what the seizures look like and how the child reacts after the seizure.

  C.   Ask if the parent/guardian wants to be called when the child has a seizure.

XV. **The child with an unexpected seizure**

  A.   If the seizure ends and the child is awake, call the parent/guardian and advise seeking a medical evaluation for the child immediately.

  B.   If the seizure does not stop, call for emergency help.

  C.   If the child becomes blue around the lips and face, call for emergency help.

  D.   If the child has difficulty breathing, call for emergency help.

BIBLIOGRAPHY

Jackson, P. & Vessey, J. (1992). *Primary care of the child with a chronic condition.* St. Louis: Mosby Year Book.

Santinilli, N., Dodson, W., & Walton, A. (1991). *Students with seizures: A manual for school nurses.* Landover, MD: Epilepsy Foundation of America.

RESOURCES

Epilepsy Foundation of America, 4351 Garden City Drive, Suite 406, Landover, MD 20785; 1-800-542-7054 or (301) 577-0100

III. CARE NEEDS

Behavior Management

Infection Control and Handwashing

Skin Care and Diapering

Nutrition

Feeding Children with Special Needs

Oral Health

First Aid for Common Child Care Incidents

Environmental Safety

Handling Principles and Techniques

Positioning and Adaptive Equipment

Child Abuse and Neglect

Observation and Recording

BEHAVIOR MANAGEMENT

I. **Classroom techniques that will benefit all children, especially children with disabilities**

   A.   Make the setting organized and stable. Minimize physical changes, and prepare children for any that are necessary.

   1.   Make daily routines consistent so children will know what will happen next.

   2.   Establish clear and consistent rules and expectations to encourage the children's understanding and cooperation.

   a.   Enforce the same rules in the same way, using the same language.
   b.   Make explanations as short and simple as possible. Don't lecture.

   3.   Cut down on the amount of stimulation in the room. Some children do better with low levels of stimulation.

   a.   Have a quiet area with a few toys and only a few wall hangings.
   b.   Do not give a child a lot of new play materials all at once. Introduce toys gradually.
   c.   Use soft music and headphones with children who benefit from the calming effect.

   4.   Keep directions simple (one or two steps). If the child does not understand, demonstrate. Children cannot comply if they do not understand what is being asked of them.

   5.   Explain rules and expectations ahead of time, and give reminders. For example, when describing an upcoming field trip, you might want to ask the children to stay on the path. If they do so, comment later, "I'm glad you're all staying on the path."

   B.   Arrange the room and provide activities at the children's level of development, as behavior is influenced by a child's developmental level. For example, children who have

trouble using or understanding language often have trouble
following directions, using words instead of hitting, and so
forth.

1.   Know each child's developmental level (cognitive,
      speech/language, and social/emotional).

2.   Make sure activities fit the child's level, especially for
      each child with special needs.

C.   Increase the amount of praise.   Praise is most powerful
      when it helps a child feel proud of himself/herself rather
      than just "minding" the caregiver.

      1.   Effective praise is sincere, specific, and given
            immediately after the desired behavior. For example:
            "I see you're sharing the markers with Erica. That's
            nice. I bet that made her happy."

      2.   When you see a child doing something you want to
            encourage, praise the child. Catch him/her being
            good!

      3.   Praise the child after good behavior to encourage the
            child to repeat that behavior.

      4.   Be as consistent as possible in noticing and praising
            appropriate behaviors.

D.   Move from one activity to another (transition) smoothly.

      1.   Keep transition time brief, and keep the children busy.

      2.   Give children notice of the next activity.   For
            example: "We'll be going in for a snack in five
            minutes."

      3.   Help the children understand your expectations.
            Rituals, or certain ways of doing things, help children
            understand what you expect.   For example, a
            lunchtime ritual may consist of putting away toys,
            sitting in a circle to sing a song, washing hands, and
            then sitting to eat lunch.

4. Recognize the child's resistance to changing activities. You might say, for example: "I'm glad you enjoyed painting today. We can do it again tomorrow, but right now it's time to clean up."

5. Assist the child with disabilities as needed to keep up with the other children. This may mean getting the child started sooner than the others.

6. Give extra help to children who have a lot of trouble with transitions. Examples:

   a. Laminate pictures of activities that are used throughout the whole day -- for example, a picture of a child picking up toys, and another picture of a child sitting with the group and listening to a story. Show these pictures and let the children know what activity is ending and what activity the child is going to do next.
   b. Give some children an object to make the transition easier. For example, allow the child to carry a book to story time.

E. Help the child feel part of the group so he/she will want to work with the group.

   1. Help the child feel safe and secure.

   2. Encourage a "family" feeling so the children develop emotional attachments to each other and to the caregiver.

F. Other ways to avoid problems

   1. Look at situations in which children misbehave to see how the activity could be changed to avoid the problems. (For example, are children left waiting too long without something to occupy them?) A child with disabilities may need additional or different changes in activity.

2.   Give children reasonable choices.

    a.   Do not ask a child to do something if he/she really does not have a choice. For example, don't say "Do you want to pick up your toys now?" when you mean "It's time to pick up your toys now."

    b.   Offer a few choices rather than free choices to narrow down possible responses. For example: "Do you want jelly or peanut butter on your toast?" instead of "What do you want on your toast?"

    c.   When a child is offered a limited choice but refuses everything or cannot choose, state the question another way. If the child still is unable to choose, make the choice for the child ("I see you want me to choose for you").

    d.   Help children learn to make choices if they don't know how. At first, cut down on the number of choices offered.

3.   Respect the child and his/her feelings, keeping in mind that a child's self-concept affects his/her behavior. A child with disabilities may have more difficulty developing a favorable self-concept.

    a.   Never make fun of or embarrass a child.

    b.   Do not give compliments that also include criticism such as, "You shared so nicely today. Why can't you always share the toys that way?"

G.   Teach children how to regulate themselves.

1.   Teach children to pay attention to their own behavior.

2.   Be sensitive to the child's feelings. Let the child know that you understand his/her feelings while helping the child to express them in an acceptable way.

    a.   Help the child identify and talk about his/her feelings.

    b.   Provide the "feeling words" for the child at first, if necessary.

3. Step in when a child's behavior becomes uncontrollable. Help the child bring his/her behavior back to a level he/she can control.

4. If a child needs a place to get control of himself/ herself, pick a place where the child has access to a few pleasant things to do. When the child feels more comfortable, return him/her to the group.

5. When children fight, separate them and talk together about better ways to respect each other and resolve differences.

6. Teach problem-solving skills for social situations.

II. **Strategies that may be adapted to individual children with challenging behaviors**

A. Choose a strategy in keeping with the child's developmental level.

B. Observe, identify, and describe the behavior.

1. Know each child's strengths and weaknesses.

2. Ask yourself if the child is capable of changing the desired behavior (such as toilet training).

3. Do not discipline or punish behaviors the child cannot control.

4. Ask yourself if the behavior is worth worrying about or is best ignored or maybe just understood.

5. Look at the specifics surrounding the behavior:

   a. Time of day.
   b. What the child does immediately before and after.
   c. How you and the other children respond to the behavior.
   d. How often the behavior happens.
   e. How long it has been a problem.

6.　Determine what is causing the behavior. The behavior is telling you something; it is a way of communicating.

7.　Change some behaviors by getting rid of what is causing them. For example, make changes within the setting.

8.　Tell the child that his/her behavior is unacceptable. Be sure young children understand what behavior is desired and what is not.

9.　Let the child know what behavior you want instead and demonstrate it if possible.

C.　Positive reinforcement

1.　Behavior is started, maintained, strengthened, or weakened by the consequences that follow. Give rewards or positive reinforcers to increase the likelihood that the behavior will be repeated.

    a.　Behaviors that are followed by positive reinforcers (rewards) tend to increase in strength or frequency.

    b.　There is no formula of reinforcement that works the same way for every child.

    c.　If a child's good behavior is strengthened through reward, the child is less likely to misbehave.

2.　Some general rules for using reinforcers effectively are as follows:

    a.　Reward good behavior immediately each time it occurs to get it going.

    b.　Be sure the reward itself is meaningful to the child. Is the reward something that makes the child feel good?

    c.　Make sure the behavior is specific enough so someone else would be able to observe it and reinforce the child.

    d.　Reward small steps in the right direction. Do not expect perfection the first few times.

       e.   Reward improvements.

       f.   Reward periodically after a behavior is well established to ensure the behavior is kept. Have a plan for reducing the frequency of reinforcement.

       g.   The first time you skip reinforcing a behavior, be sure the child is reinforced the next time the behavior occurs.

D.   Ignoring and extinction

    1.   Respond to desired behavior with a hug, smile, praise, reward, and ignore inappropriate behavior. Behaviors that do not get a response may go away (called extinction).

    2.   Do not ignore behavior that is dangerous or destructive.

    3.   When you ignore a behavior, pay *no* attention to that behavior. Do not look at or talk to the child.

    4.   When the child stops the inappropriate activity and begins an appropriate activity, praise the child.

E.   Redirection -- replacing an inappropriate form of an activity with an appropriate form of the same activity. For example, coloring on the wall with a marker is not permitted. Redirect the activity by giving the child a piece of paper to color on or replace the marker with a dry, soft paintbrush and permit the child to pretend to paint on the wall.

    1.   Provide an alternative. State what the child needs to do rather than what you want the child not to do ("Put the block on the shelf" rather than "Don't throw the block in the box").

    2.   After you have redirected the child's activity, praise the accepted behavior.

    3.   Redirect as often as necessary. It may not solve the problem the first time.

a.   This is true especially for very young children who may test the caregiver to see if the rule holds under different circumstances (for example, it's not okay to color on the wall, but maybe it's okay to color on the door).

b.   Be calm, firm, and persistent.

c.   View this "testing" as a sign of curiosity and thinking ability rather than deliberate disobedience.

F.   Setting limits (clarifies for the child both the behavior you want and the consequences if the child doesn't do this).

1.   Use when the child's behavior is inappropriate or dangerous.

2.   Steps to follow:

a.   State the rule calmly and clearly.

b.   Tell the child what to do instead, and what will happen if he/she doesn't do this.

c.   Help the child to comply by removing the child, removing toys, or other such action.

3.   Follow through:

a.   Do not repeat your request or command. This would teach the child that you do not expect him/her to comply until after the second or third request.

b.   If the child does not comply after the first request, assist him/her in doing so.

c.   Offer only choices and consequences you are willing and able to do.

G.   Natural and logical consequences

1.   Natural consequences are the automatic results of the child's own actions.

a.   For example, if a child does not eat lunch, he/she will be hungry at snack time.

        b.   Natural consequences permit children to be responsible for their own actions rather than protected from them.

  2.   Logical consequences require intervention by the caregiver.

        a.   For example, a logical consequence of a child continuing to throw sand at another child, after a reminder not to, could be to remove the child from the sand and require him/her to change activities.

        b.   Logical consequences should be applied consistently each time the problem occurs, must be logically related to the event, and must be acceptable to the caregiver.

H.   Shaping (reinforcing behaviors that are closer and closer to the desired behavior)

  1.   Use shaping to teach a new skill or to improve one that already exists.

  2.   Break down the skill into smaller, more manageable steps. Steps to follow:

        a.   Think about the behavior (or skill) you want to shape, and develop a plan, including breaking down the skill into small steps.

        b.   Reward the child for success with each step. As the child progresses from step to step, eliminate the reinforcer for the previous step.

        c.   Keep a record or time checklist noting the gradual pattern of behavior change. This also helps you to communicate in a positive way with a child's parents/guardians (for example, "Johnny hit only once today. Last week he was hitting at least three times a day. He's getting better at handling frustration").

  3.   Work on changing only one behavior at a time.

  4.   Expect setbacks. A child may master a step one day and forget it the next. In addition, an undesirable

behavior may increase when first addressing it, but then the behavior will decrease gradually while the desired behavior will increase gradually. Changing behavior takes time.

I.   Stay in charge. Be patient and maintain leadership of the interaction with the child.

1.   Avoid expressions of anger. Firmness does not require anger. You may think that anger helps get rid of your own tensions, but it does not teach the child what you think he/she should learn. Intervening earlier, before you become really angry, is better.

2.   Avoid conflict situations if possible. These usually lead to escalating power struggles.

3.   Respond to what the child is doing, not to what the child is saying. Do not lecture or argue. State simply and calmly what the problem is and what the child must do.

4.   At first, when a child is exhibiting challenging behaviors, take responsibility for your behavior and the child's behavior. Guide him/her toward a solution.

5.   Take leadership in talking with the child about his/her behaviors. Discuss and model better ways to handle the situation.

6.   Have a plan for what you expect and what your response will be to inappropriate behaviors (for example, biting). Then your response will be consistent each time, and probably more appropriate than if you react in the heat of the moment.

7.   Avoid punishment, as it distances you from the child and does not teach what you want the child to learn. It focuses the child's attention on your behavior, not the child's own behavior. You run the risk of having the child avoid you and also encouraging the child to be aggressive toward others and using the same punishment.

J.   Avoid blaming.

1.   Do not consider the child "bad" because the child behaves in ways that you or others think he/she should not. The child is not his/her actions.

2.   Label the action and your feelings, instead of the child. If you think the child has made the wrong choice, focus the child's attention and yours on the correct choice.

K.   Do not expect any child to be perfect, particularly a child facing other challenges (medical, physical, or behavioral). What might be interpreted as a child's misbehavior is really a way of communicating something.

III. **Adaptations for infants and toddlers**

A.   Infants

1.   Provide responsive care for the infant's basic needs. Anticipate needs and act before infant cries so he/she does not learn that crying gets needs met.

2.   Provide stimulation that is appropriate. An infant who has nothing interesting to look at or appealing to play with will be fussy. Likewise, with too *much* stimulation, an infant can be overwhelmed, cannot choose one thing to focus on, and becomes fussy. Learn signs of overstimulation. Infants often "shut down" and cry.

3.   Give lots of brief physical contact ("love pats") that pays attention to the infant without stopping his/her engagement in a quiet activity.

4.   Infants have short attention spans, so you can easily distract them from a behavior that you do not like and engage them in a more acceptable behavior. This is called *redirection*.

5.   Be responsible for an infant's behavior. Teach and encourage desired behaviors.

6. Couple daily routines with daily individual needs of each infant.

7. Recognize each individual infant's temperament and how the caregiving environment may be modified to match that infant's needs.

B. Toddlers

1. Distract toddlers. Utilize their short attention span and curious nature to advantage.

2. Interrupt and redirect. Head off trouble before it starts.

3. Respond to toddler's building frustration before it results in misbehavior. (This does not mean eliminating challenges, which allow the toddler to experience success and a feeling of competence.)

4. Structure activities to allow successes.

5. Be sure your rules are simple, specific, and consistent.

6. Give attention and reward good behavior without distracting the child from appropriate activity. "Catch the child being good."

7. Briefly move him/her to a quiet spot within sight of you. If toddler needs to regain control, or if he/she returns calmly, do not mention the prior behavior. Let the child start with a clean slate.

8. Ignore! If a behavior is not dangerous and is not causing a real problem in the group, just ignore it.

IV. Points to remember

A. Changing a child's behavior is not easy and takes time. There are no quick fixes, and no one "trick" works for every child. Some methods, however, will benefit all children, especially children with special needs.

B.   If what you are doing is not working, you should try something different instead of trying harder. Ask for another's input. Caregivers, teachers, and parents can easily get caught in a vicious cycle with a child and be unable to see what is happening. Another adult's observations and insight may help you see how to break the cycle.

C.   You should expect to make mistakes. We all do. Learn from them and maintain healthy, positive interactions with children.

D.   Staff members need to support each other. Working with children who have behavior problems results in a high burnout rate. Caregivers must take the time to meet with each other to share experiences and find ways to support each other.

BIBLIOGRAPHY

Brazelton, T. B. (1994). *Touchpoints: Your child's emotional and behavioral development.* Reading, MA: Addison-Wesley

Crary, E. (1993). *Without spanking or spoiling: A practical approach to toddler and preschool guidance.* Seattle: Parenting Press.

Essa, E. (1990). *A practical guide to solving preschool behavior problems,* 2d ed. Albany, NY: Delmar Publishers.

Kvigne, V., Struck, J., Englehart, E., & West, T. (1993). Education techniques for children with FAS/FAE. In J. Kleinfeld & S. Wescott (Eds.), *Fantastic Antone succeeds! Experiences in educating children with fetal alcohol syndrome.* University of Alaska Press, 323-339.

Lally, J. R., Torres, Y. L., & Phelps, P. C. (1994). Caring for infants and toddlers in groups: Necessary considerations for emotional, social, and cognitive development. *Zero to three/National Center for Clinical Infant Programs, 14*(5), 1-8.

Schmitt, B. D. (1991). *Your child's health: The parents guide to symptoms, emergencies, common illnesses, behavior & school problems.* New York: Bantam Books.

RESOURCES

Booklets available from Pro-Ed, 8700 Shoal Creek Boulevard, Austin, TX 78757-6897; 512-451-3246:

"How to Use Systematic Attention and Approval (Social Reinforcement)," by R. V. Hall and M. C. Hall.

"How to Use Planned Ignoring," by R. V. Hall and M. C. Hall.

RECOMMENDED CHILDREN'S BOOKS

Many books for young children provide opportunities for adults and children to talk about emotions and socially appropriate behaviors. Some good examples are listed below. Check for these and others at your local library or book store.

Anhott, C., & Anhott, L. (1995). *What makes me happy?* Cambridge, MA: Candlewick Press.

Berenstain, S., & Berenstain, J. (1988). *The Berenstain Bears and the bad dream.* New York: Random House.

Berenstain, S., & Berenstain, J. (1995). *The Berenstain Bears and the green-eyed monster.* New York: Random House.

Bridwell, N. (1987). *Clifford's manners.* New York: Scholastic.

Carle, E. (1977). *The grouchy ladybug.* New York: Harper & Row.

Carle, E. (1995). *The very lonely firefly.* New York: Philomel Books.

Carlson, N. (1988). *I like me!* New York: Viking Kestrel.

Carlson, N. (1994). *How to lose all your friends.* New York: Viking.

Carter, J. (editor), & Levin, J. (photographer) (1992). *Helping.* New York: Scholastic Books.

Duncan, R. (1989). *When Emily woke up angry.* New York: Barron's Educational Series, Inc.

Holy Cross School Kindergartners & Kovalcik, T. (illustrator) (1993). *What's under your hood, Orson?* Albany, NY: Scholastic Books.

Kaplan, C. (1988). *The brown bear who wasn't.* St. Louis: Milliken.

Kaplan, C. (1988). *The picky pig.* St. Louis: Milliken.

Lasky, K. (author), & McCarthy, B. (illustrator) (1993). *The tantrum.* New York: Macmillan.

Lindbergh, R. (author), and Jeffers, S. (paintings) (1987). *The midnight farm.* New York: Dial Books for Young Readers.

Mathews, J., & Robinson, F.; Natchev, A. (illustrator) (1994). *Nathaniel Willy, scared silly.* New York: Bradbury Press.

Mayer, G., and Mayer, M. (1992). *A very special critter* (A Golden Book). Racine, WI: Western Publishing Company.

Mayer, M. (1983). *I was so mad* (A Golden Book). Racine, WI: Western Publishing Company.

Pfister, M. (author), & James, J. A. (translator) (1992). *The rainbow fish.* New York: North-South Books.

Preston, E. M. (author), & Bennett, R. (illustrator) (1969). *The temper tantrum book.* New York: Scholastic Books.

INFECTION CONTROL AND HANDWASHING

I.   **Definition of infectious diseases:** contagious illnesses; can be spread from person to person.

II.   **Types of infection common in child care settings**

    A.   Respiratory tract infections. Six to eight respiratory infections per year is average for young children; children between ages 6 months and 1 year are most susceptible.

        1.   Susceptibility/complications. Some children are more likely than others to catch colds and other respiratory illnesses and also tend to have complications.

           a.   Children with:

               (1)   Down syndrome tend to have more upper respiratory infections than other children.
               (2)   Cleft palate are susceptible to ear infections.
               (3)   Poor muscle tone who cannot cough effectively are more likely to get pneumonia.
               (4)   Asthma, congenital heart disease, chronic lung disease, cystic fibrosis, and those who receive oxygen therapy or are immunosuppressed are more endangered by respiratory infections.

           b.   Efforts should be made not to expose children who are more susceptible to respiratory infections to children with respiratory illnesses.

        2.   Types of respiratory tract infections

           a.   *Common cold:* most common infectious illness; caused by viruses.

               (1)   Symptoms: sneezing, nasal discharge, congestion, fever, general malaise, headache, cough.
               (2)   Treatment: treatment of symptoms or medical attention.
               (3)   Control/prevention: spread by airborne droplets (the most common transmission mode) or by direct contact. Higher risk

in day care and preschool. More preva-
lent in winter. Children usually are
allowed to stay in the child care setting
unless they have a fever. Handwashing
is the key to prevention.

b.   *Otitis media:* recurring infection of the middle
       ear; often occurs along with an upper
       respiratory infection. Most common in
       children between 6 months and 36 months of
       age.

       (1)   Symptoms: tugging at ear or holding
             hand over ear; also may include general
             cold symptoms, fever, drainage from ear.
       (2)   Treatment: prescribed antibiotics.
       (3)   Control/prevention: not considered con-
             tagious, but accompanying respiratory
             illness may be contagious. Children
             prone to otitis media should be prevented
             from interacting with children with upper
             respiratory illnesses.

c.   *Strep throat:* infection caused by streptococcal
       bacteria.

       (1)   Symptoms: very red, sore throat that
             may be accompanied by coldlike symp-
             toms and fever.
       (2)   Treatment: antibiotic-prescribed
             therapy.[1]
       (3)   Control/prevention: children on
             medication for 24 hours are considered
             no longer contagious.

d.   *Croup:* viral infection most common in
       children between ages 3 months and 36
       months.

---

[1]   Administration of medication is generally regarded as an invasive procedure and,
      as such, is a nursing task that may be subject to regulations established by your
      State's Nursing Board. If this is the case, legislation or regulatory guidelines
      may be in place that determine whether or not and how this task may be
      delegated to a non-health-licensed individual (other than the child's parent or
      guardian). For the safety of the children, and due to the risk of personal and
      agency liability, you are urged to contact your State Board of Nursing to inquire
      about the status of delegation of invasive procedures in your state.

        (1)   Symptoms: a barking cough that often worsens at night.

        (2)   Treatment: usually at home, using cool humidifiers to moisten the air and by increasing fluid intake. Children prone to complications or having difficulty breathing may be hospitalized for treatment.

        (3)   Control/prevention: child frequently is able to return to child-care setting in 3 to 5 days.

    e.   *Whooping cough (pertussis):* a serious, contagious bacterial infection.

        (1)   Symptoms: a "whoop" sound on inhalation, with coughing spasms.

        (2)   Treatment: medical attention and prescribed antibiotics; child may have to be hospitalized.

        (3)   Control/prevention: spread by airborne respiratory droplets. DPT (diphtheria, tetanus, pertussis) vaccine given in a series beginning at 2 months of age (children immunized with partial doses of DPT are *not* immunized adequately against pertussis). Close contacts should receive preventive treatment regardless of their immunization status. Vaccine may become less protective over time, so adults and teenagers may be susceptible to pertussis and could transmit it to children, who do not have the proper immunizations.

    f.   *Pneumonia:* a potentially serious lung infection caused by viruses and bacteria; more likely to occur following an upper respiratory infection.

        (1)   Symptoms: vary with individual's age and causative agent. Usually present are increased respiratory rate, retractions, grunting, nasal flaring. Cough may not be present. Also possible: fever, chills, chest pain, nausea, vomiting.

        (2)   Treatment: medical attention and prescribed treatment regimen.

(3)   Control/prevention: children with chronic illnesses and those with poor muscle tone are more susceptible to pneumonia.   Any respiratory infection they get should be treated immediately.

g.   *H flu (Haemophilus influenza type B):*   a bacteria responsible for many illnesses, the most serious of which are meningitis and epiglottitis.

(1)   *Meningitis*: serious bacterial infection.

(a)   Symptoms: stiff neck, vomiting, irritability, lethargy (listlessness).
(b)   Treatment: immediate medical attention needed.

(2)   *Epiglottitis*:   serious bacterial infection causing swelling of epiglottis to the extent that it can block the airway; usually affects children ages 3 to 7.

(a)   Symptoms: child becomes apprehensive,   drools,   has difficulty swallowing, speaking, breathing.
(b)   Treatment: develops rapidly and requires urgent emergency care. If epiglottitis is suspected, stay with child and remain calm so as not to create further apprehension until help is secured.
(c)   Control: child usually is able to return to child care setting in 3 to 5 days.

(3)   Prevention: transmitted by respiratory droplets or direct contact. H flu vaccine is available and is recommended for all children 2 months and older and for 2-month to 5-year-old children in child care settings.

B.   Diarrheal gastrointestinal diseases: can be caused by many agents, of which the most common cause is viruses; spread by fecal-oral contamination.   Greatest risk for young children with diarrhea is dehydration.

1.   Symptoms: increase in frequency, amount, and liquid content of bowel movements; may be accompanied by nausea and vomiting.

2.   Treatment:

   a.   Adequate fluid intake in frequent small amounts
   b.   Bland diet

3.   Control/prevention: higher than average incidence of diarrhea in child care centers, especially when the same staff members are responsible for diapering infants and preparing food. Handwashing is the primary means of prevention.

C.   Rashes and skin infections

1.   *Chicken pox:*   one of the most contagious of all viruses.

   a.   Symptoms: generalized, blistering rash over the body that erupts between 11 and 20 days (but usually 14-16 days) after exposure.
   b.   Treatment: isolation, relief of symptoms, and adequate hydration.
   c.   Control/prevention: usually transmitted by respiratory droplets that disappear at about the same time the blisters crust over, or by direct contact. Contagious 1-2 days before blisters occur and until the blisters have crusted over. May return to school on the 6th day after onset of rash or if all lesions are crusted over. Anyone with the disease should not be in contact with nonimmune children or adults until the lesions have crusted over. Disease may be life-threatening for a child who has a suppressed immune system.

2.   *Impetigo:* a bacterial skin infection.

   a.   Symptoms: skin rash with a brownish-yellow (honey colored) crust, often seen around the nose and mouth but can spread to other parts of the body by direct contact.
   b.   Treatment: prescribed antibiotic therapy.

c.   Control/prevention: use clean washcloth each time you wash the child; dispose of cloth or disinfect properly. With antibiotic therapy, child may return to group child care after 48 hours.

3.   *Roseola:* viral infection usually affecting children between ages of 6 months to 36 months.

a.   Symptoms: 3 to 4 days of high fever, followed by faint, generalized rash, mainly on trunk and back of neck.

b.   Treatment: relief of symptoms (for example, fever, itching) and adequate hydration.

c.   Control/prevention: believed to be communicable only during time of fever and first day of rash.

4.   *Rubeola (measles):* a highly contagious viral disease.

a.   Symptoms: fever, cough, conjunctivitis (eye inflammation), followed by generalized rash that is most prominent on face and upper body. Lasts about 1 week.

b.   Treatment: isolation and treatment of symptoms.

c.   Control/prevention: if rubeola is suspected, isolate the child immediately. Vaccine for measles is available (first dose should be administered at 15 months of age or earlier in areas where measles is common, and second dose at either 5 years (less preferred) or 12 years (preferred) of age.

5.   *Rubella (German measles or 3-day measles):* a relatively mild viral disease, but can cause several complications to fetus if pregnant woman is infected during first 3 months of pregnancy.

a.   Symptoms: rash and fever lasting about 3 days.

b.   Treatment: isolation.

c.   Control/prevention: rubella vaccine is available and should be administered at 15 months of age as part of the MMR (measles, mumps, rubella).

6. *Fungal diaper rash:* most common in infants.

    a. Symptoms: red area on buttocks, with surrounding raw-looking areas.

    b. Treatment:

        (1) Clears only with prescription antifungal cream.

        (2) Do not use cornstarch.

        (3) Avoid use of plastic pants.

    c. Control/prevention: child may remain in child care setting if receiving treatment; rash can be transferred to others as a result of poor handwashing techniques.

D. Diseases of eyes and mouth

1. *Conjunctivitis (pink eye):* infection of clear membranes of white part of eye and inside of eyelid, caused by viruses or bacteria.

    a. Symptoms: eyes become very red, tear easily, itch or burn, may be sensitive to light, and may have a pus discharge, especially after sleeping.

    b. Treatment: most cases treated with prescribed antibiotic drops to eye. Avoid cross-contamination of other eye. If caused by herpes simplex virus and treatment is not prompt, eye could be damaged.

    c. Control/prevention: isolate children until eye drainage ceases, as most conjunctivitis is contagious.

2. *Thrush:* fungal infection of the mouth.

    a. Symptoms: tongue and inside of cheeks coated with white patches that may look like milk but do not rinse out or wipe off.

    b. Treatment: antifungal solution swabbed in mouth.[2]

    c. Control/prevention: use of sterilized nipples or pacifiers to prevent recontamination. Caregiver must use good handwashing techniques. All toys the child uses must be cleaned thoroughly.

---

[2] See footnote 1.

3. *Herpes simplex:* fever blister, cold sore.

    a. Symptoms: viral infection characterized by a blisterlike sore on mucous membranes. Lesion weeps clear fluid and slowly crusts over.
    b. Treatment: relief of symptoms.
    c. Transmitted by direct contact with saliva. Most contagious before noticeable swelling and as long as sore is present.

E. Parasites

1. *Head lice*

    a. Symptoms: scalp itching is most common symptom. Lice often are not visible, but nits (white lice eggs) can be seen attached to the hair shaft (appear like dandruff).
    b. Treatment: special prescription shampoo, followed by thorough combing of hair to remove nits.
    c. Control/prevention: highly contagious; lice are transmitted by direct contact or by contact with clothing or combs that contain the lice.

        (1) Wash all clothing and bedding in hot water or dry-clean.
        (2) Place nonwashable items in a plastic bag for 35 days.
        (3) Decontaminate stuffed animals 20 minutes in a hot dryer.
        (4) Return child to care setting after first shampoo treatment.

2. *Scabies*

    a. Symptoms: itching of the skin, particularly at night, caused by a parasite mite. May look like scratches. More prominent in skin-fold areas.
    b. Treatment: prescription lotion spread over entire body from neck down. Close contacts may be treated as a preventive measure.
    c. Control/prevention: all clothing and bedding must be washed in hot water or dry-cleaned. The child is no longer contagious 24 hours after treatment.

F. Other communicable diseases

1. *Hepatitis:* viral infection that causes inflammation of the liver; may be widespread by the time it is recognized.

   a. *Hepatitis A (HAV):* common in child care settings and easily spread

      (1) Symptoms: mild flulike symptoms in young children.
      (2) Treatment: within 10 days of known exposure, gamma globulin injection can prevent the disease; otherwise symptoms are treated throughout course of disease.

      (3) Control/prevention: spread in the feces by the fecal-oral route (fecal contamination on the hands is spread to the mouth directly or through food or toys). Adults who contract hepatitis usually are more severely ill than children.

   b. *Hepatitis B (HBV):* viral infection of the liver; usually sexually transmitted disease, so not seen often in child care settings. Can be passed from infected mother to baby during birth.

      (1) Symptoms: flulike
      (2) Treatment: symptoms are treated through course of disease; no cure available.
      (3) Control/prevention: recommended childhood immunization.

2. *Cytomegalovirus (CMV):* relatively common infection in child care populations. Peak incidence 1 to 3 years of age. Fetuses of pregnant women who are not immune are at high risk to be born with severe defects.

   a. Symptoms: few or no symptoms.
   b. Treatment: no intervention or vaccine available.

c.   Control/prevention: transmitted by direct contact with body fluids (saliva, urine, feces) and can be excreted for months after the initial infection.

III.   Preventing and controlling infectious disease

A.   Handwashing: the single most effective method of preventing infection and breaking the infection cycle. Frequent, thorough handwashing is the most effective way to curb the spread of all infectious diseases.

1.   Purposes of handwashing

a.   To remove germs from hands
b.   To prevent spread of germs to others
c.   To prevent germs from entering the body (for example, through a scratch or with food)

2.   Indications for handwashing by caregiver

a.   Important times for staff to wash hands

(1)   After arriving at the center or before the first child arrives
(2)   Before preparing, serving, or eating food
(3)   Before preparing or giving medication
(4)   After every diaper change and after helping a child with toileting
(5)   After wiping the nose of a child or caregiver's own nose
(6)   After cuddling or caring for an ill child

b.   Times for children to wash hands

(1)   After arriving at the center
(2)   If self-feeding, before eating
(3)   After using the toilet
(4)   After wiping nose, off and on when child coughs frequently and after touching any contaminated material
(5)   After coming in from outdoor play
(6)   Before handling *any* food, playing at water table, and being involved in preparation of any food items

3. Necessary equipment

    a. Sink with running water

    b. Soap

        (1) Pump-type container

            (a) Clean pumper with disinfectant daily to prevent contamination.

            (b) Empty containers weekly and clean them.

        (2) Bar soap

            (a) Provide drainage for wet soap.

            (b) To prevent bar soap from getting lost, place it in a nylon sock and tie it to faucet.

    c. For nailbrushes that can be sterilized in a dishwasher, do this daily.

    d. Manicure sticks: use disposable ones, or sterilize after each use.

    e. Use paper towels.

    f. Have basket or container that is nonabsorbent and easily cleanable for disposing of paper towels. A waste container with a lid attached to a foot pedal or a tight-fitting lid deters child from getting to waste.

4. Staff preparation

    a. Keep fingernails short and filed.

    b. Wear no jewelry except plain bands.

    c. Roll up sleeves at least 6" above wrist.

    d. Remove watch.

5. Procedure

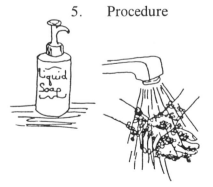

    a. Stand in front of sink. Do not lean on sink or splash water on clothing.

    b. Turn on water comfortably warm.

    c. Wet hands and lower arms.

    d. Apply soap to hands.

    e. Rub vigorously in circular movements to wash palm, back of hand, and 4" above

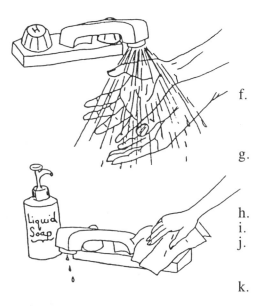

wrist of each hand. Interlace fingers and thumbs and move back and forth. Action should last at least 15 seconds.

f. Give special attention to fingernail area, using brush or orange stick to clean under fingernails.

g. Hold hands under running water to rinse arms and hands thoroughly, with fingertips pointed downward.

h. Dry with paper towel.

i. Use towel to turn off faucet.

j. Encourage students to wipe off sink so germs do not grow in standing water.

k. Discard paper towel in wastebasket.

B. Isolating sick children

1. Avoid contact between children who have respiratory infections and children who are particularly susceptible to upper respiratory diseases.

2. Avoid toy sharing between children who have respiratory infections and those who do not.

3. Be informed about exclusion policies, and enforce those policies.

4. Ideally, have an isolated area to care for children with illnesses until parent/guardian can pick up the child.

C. Toy cleaning

1. Wash toys daily with hot, soapy water. Disinfect toys with bleach or a commercial product.

2. Place toys that a child has mouthed into a container that other children cannot reach until the toys can be cleaned.

3.   Do not allow children with infectious diseases to share toys with other children.

D.   Disinfecting environmental surfaces (tables, diaper changing areas, mats for naps)

1.   Least expensive effective disinfectant solution is liquid bleach (sodium hypochlorite). Centers for Disease Control and Prevention recommend a solution of 1/4 cup bleach to 1 gallon water (1 tablespoon liquid bleach to 1 quart water; one part liquid bleach to 99 parts water). Solution should be mixed daily as it loses effectiveness after 24 hours.

2.   Clean all environmental surfaces daily, first with a cleaning solution (soapy water), then a disinfectant solution. Allow disinfectant solution to dry on surface and not be wiped off.

a.   Tables: Clean after messy play and before meals, before children arrive in the morning, and if visibly soiled.
b.   Counters and food-preparation surfaces: Clean before meals and snacks, before children arrive in the morning, and if visibly soiled.
c.   Diaper-changing areas: Cover with clean paper towels or paper covering for each child; wipe with disinfectant solution after each use. If not able to let air-dry between each use, disinfect surface and air-dry daily before children arrive.
d.   Sleeping mats: Provide a mat and sheet for each child. Clean mats weekly; disinfect and let air-dry. Wash sheets weekly.
e.   Potty chairs: Empty into toilet, clean into utility sink, and disinfect. If potty chair is cleaned in handwashing sink, disinfect sink afterward, before washing hands. Use utility gloves or disposable latex gloves to reduce spread of disease.

E.   Other recommendations

1.   All new personnel should receive handwashing demonstration.

2.   Staff members who change diapers should not prepare meals.

3.   Potty chairs should not be rinsed in sinks where food is prepared.

4.   Children with fever and those with diarrhea should be excluded from day care or isolated.

5.   Staff members should be up-to-date on their vaccinations against communicable diseases.

6.   Guidelines regarding attendance and infectious disease should apply equally to children and staff.

BIBLIOGRAPHY

American Public Health Association/American Academy of Pediatrics. (1992). *National health and safety performance standards: Guidelines for out-of-home child care programs.* Arlington, VA: National Center for Education in Maternal and Child Health.

Aronson, S. (1990). Health and safety in child care. In S. Chehrazi (Ed.), *Psychosocial issues in day care.* Washington, DC: American Psychiatric Press.

Kendrick, A., Kaufmann, R., & Messenger, K. P. (Eds.) (1991). *Healthy young children: A manual for programs (rev.).* Washington DC: National Association for the Education of Young Children.

Nahata, M. (1986). Prevention of infection by handwashing. *Child Care Newsletter, 5,* 6-11.

RESOURCES

National Association for the Education of Young Children:
1-800-424-2460 or (202) 232-8777

National Immunization Information Hotline: 1-800-232-2522

SKIN CARE AND DIAPERING

I. **Skin care**

    A.   Healthy skin is the first line of defense against invasion of bacteria that cause infections.

    B.   Children who are unable to move themselves to change positions are vulnerable to skin problems.

        1.   Many children with special needs have less awareness than other children of touch, pain, and heat or cold.

        2.   Insensitive skin is more prone to injury.

    C.   To maintain healthy skin and prevent injury:

        1.   Avoid extremes in temperature.

        2.   Prevent damage to skin from pressure caused by tight clothing or special equipment, or by being in one position for a long time.

        3.   Minimize exposure of the skin to urine and stool.

    D.   Warning signs of skin injury

        1.   Redness or other change of skin color in a specific area.

        2.   Swelling.

        3.   Changes in skin temperature.

        4.   Pain or discomfort.

        5.   Blistering.

        6.   Pressure sores (open sores from unrelieved pressure).

    E.   Caregiver's role

        1.   Prevention

            a.   Observe the child's skin frequently for warning signs.

            b.   Change an immobile child's position frequently.

            c.   Change diapers promptly when wet or soiled.

2.   Prompt treatment of:

   a.   Cuts or abrasions (cleanse and bandage as needed).
   b.   Reddened areas (change the child's position).
   c.   Pressure sores (change the child's position).

II.   Hygienic diapering

A.   Changing area.   A safe, separate table should be used specifically for changing diapers.   It must be sturdy enough to allow for the larger size of older children if they are to be changed.

B.   Frequency

   1.   Change soiled diapers promptly to prevent the child's skin from becoming irritated and breaking down.

   2.   In general, change diapers more often if a child has limited movement.

C.   Encourage intake of fluids to decrease urine concentration for less irritation of the skin.

D.   Method and procedure

   1.   Wear disposable gloves during diaper changes.[1]

   2.   Observe the urine and stool for color, odor, and amount, and record for the parent/guardian.

   3.   Observe skin in the diaper area for redness, irritating abrasions, pressure area, or rashes.   Report any indication of a developing rash or skin problem to the parent/guardian.

   4.   Clean buttocks and perineal area with warm water and a mild soap or disposable wipes (according to parent/guardian instructions).   Wipe from front to back.

   5.   Rinse and pat dry with a towel, or air dry (1-2 minutes).   Do not rub the skin.

---

[1]   Universal precautions for preventing the transmission of infectious diseases require wearing disposable gloves during diaper changes.

6.   Apply ointment to the buttocks only upon request of the parent and with written permission.[2]

7.   Disposal

a.   Dispose of soiled diaper in a *waste container* near the changing table.

b.   Place soiled clothing in a plastic bag, and send home with parent.

8.   After each use, wipe off the changing table and any area the diaper or soiled clothing came in contact with, using an effective disinfectant.

9.   After each diaper change, dispose of gloves *and* wash hands thoroughly with antibacterial soap and warm water.

E.   Special diapering conditions

1.   If prescribed or recommended, use double diapering to keep a child in a comfortable position and promote normal placement of the hips. Reuse the outer diaper if it is not soiled or wet.

2.   For children who are at higher risk for urinary tract infections, use careful diapering technique and closely observe the quality and quantity of urine. These include children with spina bifida or with spinal cord injury.

3.   For children who have casts covering the lower portion of their bodies, use special diapering techniques to prevent the cast from being soiled by urine and stool. The child's health care provider should provide special instructions.

4.   Older children

a.   Respect the child's self-esteem and privacy. Do not change the diaper in front of other children, and do not draw attention to the child's need for diapers.

---

[2] Prescription ointments are medications absorbed into the skin and should be regarded as an invasive procedure, subject to the regulations provided by your State Board of Nursing.

b.   Provide consistent assignment of personnel who give this care, if possible.

F.   General precautions

1.   Give children in diapers only washable toys.

2.   Keep children in small groups for all activities, including meals. Small groups are better than large groups for preventing the transmission of infectious diseases.

3.   If you prepare food, do not change diapers, and vice versa. The two functions should not overlap.

G.   How to use diapering time effectively

1.   For all young children and children with special needs, use diapering time to encourage children to visually track their hands or a toy to work on visual-motor skills and developmental skills.

2.   Help older children to sit by rotating them to their side and then pushing up with their hands when diapering is complete.

3.   Sing songs, use fingerplays, encourage eye contact, and elicit vocalizations or talking.

III.   Potty chair use[3]

A.   Use toilet training procedures consistent with the method used at home.

B.   Do not leave children alone on the potty chair.

C.   If necessary, secure the child on the chair or use adaptive equipment.

D.   Have the child wash his/her hands after using the potty chair.

E.   Clean and disinfect the sink and potty chair.

F.   Wash your hands thoroughly.

---

[3] Universal precautions for preventing the transmission of infectious diseases require wearing disposable gloves when handling soiled potty equipment.

BIBLIOGRAPHY

Boyington, R. W., Dunn, E. S., and Stephens, G. R. (1994). *Manual of ambulatory pediatrics*. Glenview, IL: Scott Foresman & Co.

Farrington, E. (1992). Diaper dermatitis. *Pediatric Nursing, 18*(1), 81-82.

NUTRITION

I. **Definition.** According to the American Medical Association, nutrition is the science of food, the nutrients therein, their action, interaction and balance in relation to health and disease and the process of metabolism by which the organism ingests, digests, transports, utilizes, and excretes food substances.

II. **Fundamentals of nutrition**

A. The body uses nutrients to

1. produce energy in a process called *metabolism,* and

2. maintain regulatory functions.

B. The unit of measurement is the *calorie;* the number of calories a child needs depends on size, amount of physical activity, rate of growth, and age.

C. Good nutrition is essential for normal physical growth and development of the intellectual, social, educational, and behavioral skills of the growing child.

D. Good nutrition begins before the child is born. Mothers with poor nutrition during their pregnancy increase their risk of delivering a low birth weight, premature, or stillborn infant.

III. **Classifications of nutrients**

A. Carbohydrates

1. Supply up to half of the energy requirements of infants, toddlers, and young children

2. The two main types

a. *Simple carbohydrates:* sugars found in fruits and milk; a source of quick energy
b. *Complex carbohydrates:* starches and fiber found in cereals and vegetables. Starches are a source of slowly released energy, and fiber provides bulk to the stool

B. Fats

1. Necessary for growth and healthy skin and also insulate against heat loss

    2.   Found in vegetable oils, animal fats, dairy products, and breast milk

C.   Proteins

    1.   The body breaks down proteins into amino acids and nitrogen.

        a.   Amino acids are involved in building new tissue, hormones, enzymes, and antibodies.
        b.   Nitrogen maintains existing tissue health.

    2.   Foods high in protein include meat, fish, poultry, eggs, and dairy products.

D.   Vitamins

    1.   Two types of vitamins

        a.   Water-soluble: cannot be stored in the body, so should be taken in daily
        b.   Fat-soluble: can be stored in the body

    2.   Specific functions of various vitamins are

        a.   Vitamin A: keeps skin healthy and aids in night vision
        b.   Vitamin B complex: helps release energy from food
        c.   Vitamin C: keeps connective tissue healthy and helps the body fight infection
        d.   Vitamin D: helps the body absorb and use calcium for bone development and neuromuscular activity
        e.   Vitamin E: protects body tissues
        f.   Vitamin K: helps with blood clotting

    3.   Found in all types of food, including fruits, vegetables, dairy products, cereals, grains, seeds, beans, oil, meats, and fish

E.   Minerals

    1.   The main classifications are

        a.   Macrominerals (major): seven minerals the body needs daily: calcium, phosphorus, potassium, sulfur, sodium chloride (salt), magnesium.

b. Microminerals or trace minerals: those the body requires in very small amounts: iron, zinc, copper, manganese, selenium, fluoride, iodine, chromium, molybdenum.

2. Minerals help build healthy bones and teeth, transport oxygen, help control the heart, help blood clot, involved in enzyme systems, and promote growth and healing.

3. Minerals are found in dairy products, meats, breads, and cereals.

F. Water

1. Second only to oxygen as being essential for life

2. Comprises 60% to 70% of body weight

3. Regulates body temperature, lubricates body parts, and is an essential part of the body's transportation system

IV. **Healthy nutrition by age classification**

A. Infants

1. Birth to 4 months

a. Milk in the form of mother's breast milk or a commercially prepared formula will provide infants under 4-6 months with all their nutritional requirements.
b. Fluoride and vitamin D supplements usually are added to the breastfeeding diet.

2. 4-6 months

a. Strained and semi-solid foods are introduced gradually into infants' diets.
b. Cereal fortified with iron is introduced first, followed by fruits, vegetables, and meats.
c. Foods are introduced one at a time for 3-4 days, with at least two between-meal snacks, watching for signs of any sensitivities or allergies.
d. Semi-solid foods are added gradually to infants' diets as they develop are able to handle food that requires more chewing.

3.   6 months to 1 year

    a.   Children in this age group can be given three meals per day with between-meal snacks.

    b.   Breast milk or formula can be offered in a cup as well as the bottle; intake should not be more than 24 ounces in 24 hours.

B.   Toddlers (1-3 years)

1.   Toddlers should be encouraged to eat a wide variety of foods.

2.   They should be encouraged to give up the bottle, drink from a cup, and feed themselves.

3.   Toddlers' appetite begins to decrease, and often they refuse to eat regular meals.

4.   At least 3-4 hours should be allowed between meals, as "grazing" suppresses feelings of hunger and results in inadequate nutrient intake.

5.   Foods to avoid include small, hard candy, nuts, grapes, hot dogs, popcorn, and other foods a toddler could choke on.

C.   3-5 years

1.   Rate of growth decreases, and so does appetite, although appetite increases slowly again when the child gets closer to school age.

2.   Children are independent — ask for and seek food, drink from a cup rather than a bottle, feed themselves without help, and prepare simple foods such as cereal with milk.

3.   They often have food jags, eating the same food constantly.

4.   Consuming five or six meals a day is common.

5.   Food preferences include carbohydrate-rich foods such as cereal, grains, and potatoes. Other food preferences are sweets, dairy products, and juice. They tend to dislike cooked vegetables, mixed dishes, and liver.

6.   Milk intake decreases to 1-2½ cups per day.

V.   **Common nutritional concerns of children with special needs**

A.   Feeding a child involves much more than simply supplying nutrients; it also involves strong emotions for both child and caregiver. Mealtime offers an excellent opportunity for the child to develop physically, mentally, emotionally, socially, and educationally. It also is an ideal setting for the child to develop self-esteem.

B.   The feeding relationship can be altered when

1.   a child rejects food,

2.   the child cannot take in the food, and/or

3.   the child cannot take in enough food for growth and development.

C.   Feeding problems are defined as the inability or refusal to eat certain foods because of neuromuscular dysfunctions, obstructive lesions, or psychological factors. Delayed development of a feeding skill often has both a physical and a psychological basis.

1.   The neuromuscular dysfunctions of hypotonia (too little muscle tone) or hypertonia (too much muscle tone) associated with cerebral palsy often result in sucking, chewing, and swallowing difficulties.

2.   An obstructive malformation, often present in children with cleft lip or cleft palate, can result in sucking and swallowing difficulties.

3.   Psychological factors present in children with autism may lead to refusal of food, dehydration, and malnutrition.

D.   Metabolic and digestive process disorders

1.   In metabolic disorders certain enzymes that are necessary to break down food into nutrients may be absent or reduced greatly. If left untreated, the child will become malnourished and may suffer brain damage.

2.   Examples of metabolic and digestive conditions are:

    a.   *Cystic fibrosis:*   Children with CF do not secrete the pancreatic enzyme necessary for the body to absorb fats and fat-soluble vitamins. They must take pancreatic enzymes as a supplement.

    b.   *Celiac disease:*   Children with celiac disease react to (like an allergy) the gluten in cereal grains and flour.   They must take enzyme supplements and remove gluten from their diet.

    c.   *PKU:*   Children with PKU lack the enzyme needed to break down phenylalanine, found in infant formulas and other dairy products.   If left undiagnosed and untreated, these children will develop severe retardation, hyperactivity, and seizures.   All newborns are tested for PKU.

    d.   *Short bowel syndrome/GI dysfunction*: Children with GI dysfunction are unable to digest and absorb nutrients. Thus, intravenous or gastrointestinal tube feeding is necessary to sustain growth.

E.   Obesity[1]

    1.   Children with Down syndrome, children who receive assisted ventilation, and those with other developmental disorders that result in decreased activity are at higher risk for becoming obese.

    2.   Obesity increases the child's risk for developing heart disease, high blood pressure, and diabetes.

    3.   Treatment for obesity usually includes behavior management, controlled calorie intake, and increased activity.

F.   Constipation

    1.   Lack of activity in children with special needs increases the risk for constipation, which often reduces the child's appetite.

---

[1] Children with muscular dystrophy and cerebral palsy, although inactive, may have difficulty with sucking and swallowing, which often results in failure to thrive, not obesity.

      2. Constipation is best prevented by adding high-fiber foods and extra fluids to the diet. The child's physician may prescribe laxatives and suppositories.

G. Problems with long-term drug therapy

      1. Medications such as anticonvulsants, tranquilizers, stimulants, diuretics, and laxatives often affect the absorption of vitamins, retention of electrolytes, and development of bones and teeth. Medications also may increase or decrease appetite.

      2. Children with epilepsy who take anticonvulsant drugs often develop problems with sore mouth and hyperplasia of the gums.

      3. Laxatives prescribed for constipation can cause loss of potassium from the body.

      4. Children with attention deficit disorder sometimes are prescribed stimulants such as Ritalin that depress their appetite and reduce their rate of growth.

      5. Chemotherapy treatments for children with cancer cause loss of appetite, vomiting, and diarrhea.

      6. Nutritional counseling usually is indicated for children with drug-nutrient interactions.

H. Feeding relationship problems

      1. Inappropriate feeding practices, nutritional misinformation, lack of knowledge in food preparation, and difficulty setting limits around food and feedings can lead to nutritional deficits in children with special needs.

      2. The feeding relationship between the caregiver and the child may become troubled.

          a. The caregiver may overfeed a child, thinking food is one of the child's few pleasures.
          b. The caregiver may offer foods that are easiest for a child to eat but that delay the child's developmental progress.

3.   Some caregivers are vulnerable to nutritional misinformation (fad diets, megavitamin therapy, supplements of various origins) that may affect their thinking and actions in regard to feeding children.

I.   Failure to thrive (FTT)

1.   "Failure to thrive" describes a group of symptoms present in malnourished children below the 5th percentile for height and weight. These children fail to gain weight normally, often are developmentally slow, and have feeding problems, sleep disturbances, and a lack of interest in their environment.

2.   Possible organic contributing factors include metabolic disorders, genetic defects, prematurity, and prenatal malnutrition.

3.   Nonorganic risk factors include families that are socially isolated, overwhelmed parents, stress, and depression in the mother-infant relationship. Also, families may be poor or homeless.

4.   Intervention and treatment

a.   Treatment utilizes a team approach with physicians, nutritionists (R.D.), social workers, and nurses.
b.   Malnutrition is treated by improving the child's diet (increasing the child's caloric and protein intake), and in some circumstances supplementing calories with tube feedings.
c.   Attempts should be made to strengthen the feeding relationship between the child and the parent/guardian, improve the child's feeding schedule, and provide emotional and social support for the parents.

VI.   Nutritional assessment

A.   The nutritional status of the child with special needs may be assessed by

1.   taking a health and feeding history from the child's parent/guardian,

2.   observing feeding of the child,

3. keeping a 24-hour intake record or a 3-day diet diary for the child,

4. taking growth measurements: height, weight, head circumference, skinfold thickness; doing a developmental assessment on the child,

5. using laboratory testing to assess how the child's body is utilizing the nutrients, and/or

6. assessing the psychosocial and economic status of the family, taking into account religious and cultural food preferences.

B. This nutritional assessment is done by a registered dietitian (R.D.). Following the assessment, the R.D. often works with an interdisciplinary team to plan a program that meets the child's nutritional needs. This interdisciplinary team may include

1. physician,

2. nurse,

3. dental specialist,

4. speech pathologist,

5. pharmacist,

6. neurologist, and

7. physical therapist (PT)/occupational therapist (OT).

BIBLIOGRAPHY

Bailey, D. B., Harms, T., & Clifford, R. M. (1983). Social and educational aspects of mealtimes for handicapped and non-handicapped preschoolers. *Topics in early childhood special education, 3*(2), 19-32.

Batshaw, M. & Perret, Y. M. (1992). *Children with handicaps: A medical primer*. Baltimore: Paul H. Brooks Publishing.

Bithoney, W. (1989). Failure to thrive. *Early Childhood Update, 5*(3), 1.

Morris, S. E., & Klein, M. D. (1987). *Prefeeding skills: A comprehensive resource for feeding development.* San Antonio, TX: Therapy Skill Builders.

Pipes, P. L. (Ed.) (1989). *Nutrition in infancy and childhood* (4th ed.). St. Louis: Times Mirror/Mosby.

Satter, E. (1987). *How to get your kid to eat: But not too much.* Palo Alto: Bull Publishing.

Smith, M. A. H., Connolly, B., McFadden, S., Nicrosi, C., Nuckolls, L., & Russell, F. *Management of a child with a handicap. A guide for professionals.* Memphis: University of Tennessee Center for the Health Sciences, Child Development Center.

RESOURCES

Consumer Nutrition Hotline: 1-800-366-1655

National Center for Nutrition and Dietetics, 216 West Jackson Blvd., Suite 800, Chicago, IL 60606; (312) 899-0040, ext. 4653

• *Recommended Dietary Allowances (RDA).* National Academy of Sciences, Government Printing Office, Washington, DC

National Maternal and Child Health Clearing House, 8201 Greensboro Drive, Suite 600, McLean, VA 22102; (703) 821-8955, ext. 265

• *Starting Early: A Guide to Federal Resources and Child Health*

Regional Nutrition Consultant, Public Health Service Regional Office

Local Office of State Department of Health: Nutritional Services

State WIC Program

FEEDING CHILDREN WITH SPECIAL NEEDS

I. **Why eating is important**

    A.   Nutrition affects growth and learning.

    B.   Infant feeding develops muscles in the face and mouth that also are required for speech.

    C.   Untreated eating difficulties may result in dental or facial abnormalities.

    D.   Eating involves interaction between the child and parent/guardian/caregiver that affects the child psychologically and socially.

II. **The process of eating**

    A.   The jaw and tongue move rhythmically.

    B.   The lips close around the nipple or spoon to keep food or liquid in the mouth.

    C.   The roof of the mouth moves to prevent food or liquid from entering the nose.

    D.   The tongue moves the food or liquid toward the back of the throat, triggering a swallowing reflex.

III. **Oral reflex development: Normal infants**

    A.   Oral reflexes set the stage for us to learn to drink and eat.

        1.   Drinking fluids starts when the infant is born.

        2.   The rooting reflex helps an infant find a nipple.

    B.   Some oral reflexes disappear as the child develops. For example, the rooting reflex is present in a newborn and not in a 6-month old. Some developmental reflexes are designed by nature to prepare an immature nervous system for controlled, voluntary movement. As voluntary motor control develops, the reflex becomes integrated and is no longer needed.

    C.   Other oral reflexes such as swallowing and gagging are lifelong.

D.   Oral reflexes essential to motor development and control include

    1.   suckling (the most primitive oral reflex),

    2.   sucking (advancement of suckling to include swallowing and breathing),

    3.   biting,

    4.   chewing, and

    5.   swallowing.

E.   The biting and chewing reflexes help the growing infant learn to eat solid foods.

    1.   At around 3-5 months of age, a normal infant bites as a reflex when a finger or a spoon is placed between the upper and lower gums.

    2.   At around 7 months of age, the infant starts to chew.

        a.   Chewing begins with a vertical rotation of the mouth.
        b.   The tongue moves toward the front of the mouth or to the right or left side of the mouth.
        c.   Eventually the child uses "rotary chewing" (switching food from side to side within the mouth while keeping the lips closed, as most adults do).

IV.   Oral reflex development: Children with disabilities

A.   Feeding problems include

    1.   drooling;

    2.   chewing;

    3.   difficulty with tongue movements; and

    4.   difficulty with sucking, chewing, and swallowing.

B.   Possible reasons for feeding difficulties

    1.   Prematurity or medical problems may affect strength.

2.   The coordination of breathing and eating may be affected by immature lung development.

3.   Some babies and young children become upset when anything comes near their mouth.

4.   Abnormalities of the mouth, tongue, or throat may be present.

5.   A neurological problem may be present that makes eating difficult.

6.   Some children have a nervous system that is too easily aroused.

7.   Muscle tone (varying from too tight to too floppy) may make eating difficult.

V.   Observation of feeding

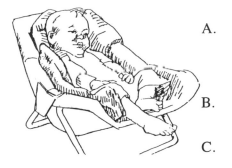

A.   The child's mother and the therapist are the best sources for the best way to feed a specific child.

B.   First the child has to be positioned and helped to relax.

C.   The child's head should be kept in a mid-line position.

Positioning a baby in an infant seat

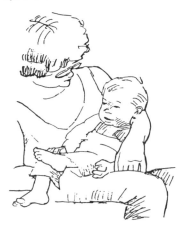

Positioning a child with muscle problems

D. The meal should be as positive an experience as possible.

    1. The food should include several tastes or textures the child likes.

    2. The atmosphere should be pleasant.

    3. Nonpreferred foods should be introduced carefully.

    4. The person feeding the child should smile and talk to the child to make the child feel safe, loved, and contented.

VI. Positioning children with muscle problems

A. Correct positioning in general:

    1. Bend the child's hips and knees.

    2. Place the child's arms forward.

    3. Place the child's head slightly forward in the body's mid-line.

    4. Offer the spoon at mid-line.

B. If a child's legs "scissor" across each other:

    1. Increase support under the child's thighs to help the legs by lifting your leg.

    2. Put a roll under the child's thighs to flex the hips.

    3. Hold the child with one leg bent more than the other and the legs separated.

    4. Place a small roll between the child's legs.

C. If a baby is overly sensitive about touch and does not like to be held while eating:

    1. Swaddle the child with hips flexed and arms forward.

    2. Place the child in an infant seat, making sure the arms and head are forward and the hips and knees are bent.

        a. Use towel rolls to keep the child's head and arms forward or to separate legs.

b. If the child's legs flop outward, use rolls under the knees or on the outside of the thighs.

c. Do not prop the bottle while baby is an infant seat because

(a) it increases the danger of choking, and
(b) the baby needs to see and hear you.

3. Use a special chair with the following characteristics:

a. It should have a footrest to support the child's feet.
b. The chair back should be high enough to support the child's head and neck.
c. The child's pelvis should be placed at the back of the chair.
d. A tray may help to support the child's arms.
e. Padding may be used to keep the child's arms and legs forward.
f. Padding between the knees can prevent scissoring.
g. Each chair should have a safety strap at the pelvis to fit low across the hips and keep the child's pelvis back into chair.

VII. Adaptive equipment

A. Different kinds of nipples are available commercially, and the health professional involved should recommend what is best for the individual child.

B. Various spoons are available.

1. Spoons with shallow bowls are best for children who have difficulty with lip muscles.

2. Different-shaped handles are available for toddlers with coordination problems.

3. Spoons with blunt ends might be used with children who have an overactive bite reflex.

4. Brittle plastic spoons (and cups) could shatter, and an uncoated metal spoon could cut the gums.

C. A cutaway cup allows the caregiver to see the level of liquid in the cup and does not require the child to tip the head back as far.

VIII. Feeding techniques

    A.   Positioning

        1.   Sit directly in front of the child, and offer the spoon at mid-line.

        2.   Keep your face at the child's eye level so the child will not have to look up, which might cause arching of the back and make it more difficult to eat.

        3.   Bring the spoon straight to the child's mouth.

    B.   Encourage the child to remove the food from the spoon with the lips. Do not scrape food off on roof of the mouth or on the upper teeth as this can cause arching, gagging, and tongue thrust.

        1.   Rest the spoon on the lower lip and wait for the child to open his/her mouth.

        2.   When the mouth opens, move the spoon in and wait for the mouth to close.

        3.   If necessary, press down on the upper lip gently to help the mouth to close.

        4.   Be sure the child's head is tipped down.

        5.   Use a spoon with a shallow bowl.

        6.   Give as few verbal cues as possible.

    C.   When the bite reflex is triggered and the jaws clamp shut hard, do not pull on the spoon; wait until the jaws relax.

        1.   To help prevent the bite reflex, position the child with hips bent, feet supported, and arms forward.

        2.   When giving a drink, rest the cup on the child's bottom lip without using pressure and without touching the teeth.

    D.   Textures

        1.   If thickened liquids are easier for an infant to swallow:

            a.   Add baby cereal to formula.

      b.   Add yogurt to milk.

      c.   Add applesauce to apple juice.

      d.   Offer fruit nectars that are naturally thick.

2.   If a child does not tolerate the combination of smooth and textured foods in the mouth at the same time (such as soup or stew):

      a.   Remove the textured food from the liquid and present one consistency at a time.

      b.   Puree different foods together.

      c.   Introduce foods with different textures slowly when the child is ready.

3.   Rate of feeding

      a.   If a child needs a longer time to eat (and may hold food in the mouth for a long time):

           (1)   Be patient; *expect* to take longer than normal.

           (2)   Feed the child slowly, with small bites.

      b   To expedite feeding and thereby prevent boredom or frustration:

           (1)   Introduce new tastes or textures at the beginning of the meal when the child is hungry.

           (2)   Give toddlers small, frequent meals.

           (3)   Offer a nutritious snack halfway between meals.

4.   Jaw control techniques: Use under the direction of the health professional familiar with the child.

IX.   Ways to make feeding easier

A.   Respect the child's natural rhythms, and watch for cues.

1.   Make sure the child is awake, alert, and hungry before feeding.

2.   If a baby is difficult to arouse when it is time to eat, unwrap and pat the baby gently.

3.   If a child does not give any cues, initiate feeding on schedule.

B.   Look for signs that the child may need to take a break in eating:

1.   crying, while pulling away;

2.   moving the arms or legs, or both, vigorously;

3.   turning the head or eyes away or pushing the food away; or

4.   falling asleep.

C.   If the baby has trouble sucking rhythmically, try rocking or playing music with the same rhythm.

D.   If mucus builds up, allow the child a break for several minutes so he/she can swallow the mucus and clear the airway.

E.   If a toddler doesn't like to have things near the mouth, expose the toddler to new smells, tastes, and textures.

1.   Put a little pureed fruit or peanut butter on a toy; let the child smell it and touch it to the lips.

2.   Offer finger foods around mealtime or snacktime.

3.   Put mashed potatoes or pudding on the child's hands, and encourage the child to put his/her hands into the mouth.

X.   Preventing distractions

A.   Turn the lights down and TV off.

B.   Send others into another room.

C.   To minimize visual distractions, turn high chair toward a blank wall.

D.   Avoid giving *too much* attention, but keep the child in sight for safety reasons.

XI.   Safety measures

A.   Feed babies in an upright or slightly reclined position to prevent choking.

    B.   Do not give young children foods they can choke on such as

        1.   raw vegetables, raw apples, grapes;

        2.   nuts, raisins, popcorn, chips; and

        3.   small pieces of hot dog.

    C.   Be alert for signs of choking including

        1.   a wet cough or gurgling after swallowing,

        2.   widening of the eyes, and

        3.   gagging or turning blue.

XII. **Behavior problems**

    A.   Avoid "battles" over eating, as it is one thing the child can control — and win.

    B.   Praise the child for behaving well and trying to eat.

    C.   Be consistent in how and where the child is fed, including a consistent meal schedule, position, and surroundings.

XIII. **Professional involvement**

    A.   Feeding problems require a health plan developed by a professional.

    B.   Progress should be monitored regularly over the long term.

    C.   The child's program should be monitored to adapt to changes.

BIBLIOGRAPHY

Fisher, A., Murray, E., & Bundy, A. (1991). *Sensory integration: Theory and practice.* Philadelphia, PA: F. A. Davis.

Geralis, E. (Ed.) (1991). *Children with cerebral palsy: A parent's guide.* Woodbine House.

Hill, A. S., & Rath, L. (1993). The care and feeding of the low-birth-weight infant. *Journal of Perinatal & Neonatal Nursing, 6*(4), 56-68.

Klein, M. D., & Delaney, T. A. (1994). *Feeding and nutrition for the child with special needs: Handouts for parents.* San Antonio, TX: Therapy Skill Builders.

Norris, M. G., & Hill, C. S. (1994). Nutritional issues in infants and children with congenital heart disease. *Critical Care Nursing Clinics of North America, 6*(1), 153-163.

Oetter, P., Richter, E. W., & Frick, S. M. (1993). *M.O.R.E.: Integrating the mouth with postural and sensory functions.* Hugo, MN: PDP Press.

Wilbarger, P., & Wilbarger, J. L. (1991). *Sensory defensiveness in children: An intervention guide for parents and other caretakers.* Santa Barbara, CA: Avanti Educational Programs.

Wolf, L. S., & Glass, R. P. (1992). *Feeding and swallowing disorders in infancy: Assessment and management.* San Antonio, TX: Therapy Skill Builders.

ORAL HEALTH

I. Oral/dental development

A. Tooth eruption, or teething, varies widely in children, especially those with developmental delays or disabilities.

1. Teeth actually begin to develop when a fetus is only about 5 weeks old.

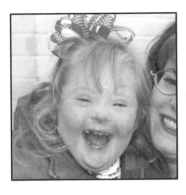

Normal tooth eruption

2. The first tooth usually erupts around 6 months of age.

3. If general development is delayed, tooth eruption also may be delayed; this may delay speech sounds and interfere with correct feeding patterns.

4. Teething can be somewhat painful and cause the child to be cranky or to drool a lot.

B. Abnormal tooth development is most often observed as small pits or lines on the teeth, discoloration, or a difference in size or shape.

1. Most of these problems are not serious and probably don't require treatment.

2. Rare cases involve all the teeth, and may require extensive treatment by a dental specialist.

C. Abnormal jaw or face development can result in crowded or malpositioned teeth or varying spaces between teeth.

1. Some of these problems can be helped by orthodontics or other types of dental treatment.

2. Major abnormalities such as cleft palate may cause respiratory, speech, and appearance problems.

3. If thumbsucking and use of a pacifier continue beyond age 5, the teeth may begin to take on abnormal positions.

251

D. Delays or dysfunction involving the tongue or oral reflexes are common in children with developmental delays.

   1. Some of these problems may interfere with dental growth and development.

   2. Some of these problems lead to retention of food in the mouth.

   3. More serious problems include choking, aspiration, and excessive gagging.

   4. Proper nursing habits help develop facial muscles and bones.

II. Common oral conditions and diseases

A. Oral infections

   1. Gum tissues are normally pink and moist and free of lumps or lesions.

   2. Infections are caused by changes in bacteria in the mouth. Common types are

      a. yeast infection (candida).
      b. herpetic lesions (cold sores).

   3. Children who have been sexually abused may have other infections in the mouth.

   4. Episodes of oral infections may be precipitated by other illnesses that challenge the immune system.

B. Gingivitis

   1. Gum tissues around the teeth generally are firm, pink, and free of sores.

   2. Cells in the gum tissues require the same adequate nutrients as other body cells.

   3. Gingivitis is characterized by inflammation, redness, and puffiness.

   4. Gingivitis can be caused by

      a. erupting teeth (will subside after the teeth have come in), or

           b.   an infection that goes away only after removing the bacterial irritant by brushing.

    5.   Children with compromised immune systems (such as HIV-positive) or connective tissue disorders (such as Down syndrome) may have severe types of gingivitis at an early age.

    6.   Breathing through the mouth can cause drying of gum tissues and aggravate gingivitis.

    7.   Early diagnosis and treatment of gingivitis can prevent later damage to the tissues supporting the teeth.

C.   Dental caries (dental decay)

    1.   Certain bacteria cause teeth to become infected and to demineralize, usually appearing as white chalky areas or as brown spots or craters.

    2.   Bacteria usually are transmitted to the child by family members through kissing or sharing eating utensils or food.

    3.   Causes include

           a.   prolonged breastfeeding or bottlefeeding with milk, soda pop, or other liquid containing sugar or acids that promote bacterial growth;
           b.   diet of foods high in carbohydrates that remain in the mouth for a long time; and
           c.   frequent vomiting.

4. Infection can spread to the nerve of the tooth or surrounding tissues causing an abscess.

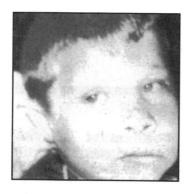

a. Usually red or white spongy bump on the tissue near the infected tooth.

b. Sometimes face will swell near the area.

Swollen face caused by dental infection
Courtesy of Mary Beth Kinney,
Indian Health Service, Keizer, OR

5. Decay usually is not painful until it reaches an advanced stage and infects the nerve.

D. Oral trauma

1. Trauma could consist of facial or intraoral lacerations, bites, fractures, burns, or knocked out teeth.

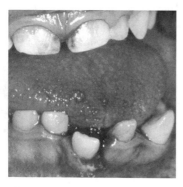

2. Causes include child abuse, falls, accidents, hot or sharp foods or objects, chewing on electrical cords.

3. Some types are mild and will heal quickly; others require prompt professional attention.

4. Early treatment might prevent later problems in developing oral structures.

Displaced tooth from oral injury
Courtesy of Lucille Adelstein Katz,
Region II Public Health Service, New York, NY

III.   Special care needs

A.   Physical limitations

1.   Children with poor motor coordination (such as with cerebral palsy and muscular dystrophy) may be unable to clean their own teeth adequately, making them dependent on others for plaque removal.

2.   Some children are unable to chew or move their tongue properly, interfering with the natural cleaning action of the tongue, cheek, and lip muscles; this leads to retaining food in the mouth.

B.   Special diets

1.   If the child has difficulty chewing and swallowing and soft or pureed food is served, it tends to be retained in the mouth longer.

2.   Children who need help drinking may take in less fluids and not wash away food particles and plaque.

3.   Eating sugary food often, using foods for behavioral reinforcers, snacking without brushing, and sleeping with a bottle can increase the chances for tooth decay.

C.   Medications

1.   Some seizure medications may cause enlarged gums, which can interfere with chewing, speech, and appearance and can lead to plaque retention and gum disease.

2.   Drugs used to control muscle activity may decrease saliva flow that usually helps protect teeth against dental decay.

3.   Some medications use syrup or sugar as sweeteners; these also can cause tooth decay if left on the teeth without rinsing the mouth.

IV.   Preventive measures and parent communication

A.   To ease discomfort from teething, let the child suck on a cold, smooth, hard object such as a teething ring.

B.   Check the temperature and consistency of foods to prevent burns, lacerations, choking, and aspiration.

C.   If a child wears a helmet for safety purposes because of seizures, consider adding a mouthguard bar.

D.   Discourage prolonged breastfeeding or bottlefeeding to entertain or quiet the child.

E.   Wash or clean the child's mouth with water after bottlefeeding or breastfeeding.

F.   Rinse or clean the child's mouth after snacks and meals.

G.   Try to not use foods as behavioral reinforcers as they can cause tooth decay and loss of appetite.

H.   If a child has a bite reflex, use a soft mouth prop to keep the mouth open while brushing the teeth.

I.   Be aware that even children who are tube-fed or have gastrostomies need their mouths cleaned, as bacteria are still present and can cause infections.

J.   Use only a pea-sized amount of toothpaste, and try not to let the child swallow the paste.

K.   With regard to fluoride:

1.   Use toothpaste containing fluoride to protect the teeth from dental decay.

a.   If the paste is too foamy, pour some fluoride rinse in a cup, dip the brush in the cup and brush with the rinse.
b.   Use only a small amount and try to prevent swallowing.

2.   Ask how much fluoride is in the water source where the child usually gets drinking water.

        a.   The dentist or physician may prescribe fluoride drops or tablets with or without vitamins if fluoride levels are deficient.

        b.   The fluoride content of bottled water varies and may not be noted on the label.

L.   Do not share toothbrushes. Store them separately so they can air-dry. Do not put them in the dishwasher. If children do accidentally share brushes, get them new ones.

M.   If indicated, suggest to parents/guardians that they ask their dentist about dental sealants for the pits and fissures of teeth, the parts most susceptible to decay. They usually are placed on the back permanent teeth, but sometimes are used for primary teeth.

V.   First aid for oral injuries.

A.   Minor injuries happen frequently during childhood, most often from falls.

B.   Although many injuries cannot be prevented, some can through appropriate supervision and safe practices

C.   For lacerations, cuts, or embedded debris:

      1.   Control bleeding.

      2.   Wash gently.

      3.   Check for fractured, chipped, or knocked-out teeth so child won't choke on the fragments.

D.   If tooth is knocked out:

      1.   Find the tooth and put it in a glass of milk. Do not try to reinsert a baby tooth in child's mouth.

      2.   Clean any debris from child's mouth and go immediately to the dentist. Depending on the child's age and other factors, the dentist may not try to reinsert a primary tooth but might if it's a permanent tooth.

      3.   If swelling is present, apply a cold compress (towel around some ice cubes).

      4.   Don't place aspirin on any area in the mouth that hurts, because aspirin can cause a chemical burn.

VI. **Teaching children to brush**

  A. Try to let the child brush as much of the mouth as possible while you help guide the position or motion of the brush.

  B. Make sure the brush has soft bristles and is small enough for the child's mouth.

  C. Make oral care as pleasant as possible. Play music, sing, talk softly, and give frequent encouragement.

  D. Do not try to teach children of this age how to floss.

  E. Adapt a toothbrush for a child who can't grasp a brush (see Figure 1, page 261).

  F. Refer to the steps in brushing teeth shown in Figure 2, page 262.

  G. Consider the helpful positions shown in Figure 3, page 263.

  1. Always support the child's head.

  2. Protect clothes from splatters.

  3. Make sure you can see inside the child's mouth.

  4. If more than one child is involved, use latex or vinyl gloves. Wash hands and change gloves between children.

BIBLIOGRAPHY

Entwistle, B. (1984). Private practice preventive dentistry for the special patient. *Special care in dentistry, 4*(6), 246-252.

Entwistle, B. A., & Casamassimo, P. S. (1981). Assessing dental health problems of children with developmental disabilities. *Journal of Developmental and Behavioral Pediatrics, 2*(3), 115-121.

Pinkham, J. R., et al. (1988). *Pediatric dentistry: Infancy through adolescence* (pp. 149-156, 171-182.) Philadelphia: W. B. Saunders.

RESOURCES

Academy of Dentistry for the Handicapped, 211 East Chicago Avenue, Chicago, IL 60611; 1-800-621-8099, ext. 2660

American Dental Association, Catalog Order Department, 211 East Chicago Avenue, Chicago, IL 60611; 1-800-947-4746

Pamphlets:

- W177: Your Child's Teeth
- W110: Your Child's First Visit to the Dentist
- W216 The Developing Smile
- Dental Care for Special People

American Dental Hygienist Association, Order Department, 444 North Michigan Avenue, Suite 3400, Chicago, IL 60611; 1-800-243-ADHA

"Preventing Baby Bottle Tooth Decay" (instructional flipchart and two pads of give-away cards with primary message)

American Society of Dentistry for Children, 875 North Michigan Avenue, Suite 4040, Chicago, IL 60611-1901; 1-800-637-ASDC

Pamphlets:

- Baby's Bright Smile
- Baby Teeth and Beyond
- Beyond Your Child's Smile
- Snack-n-Good Foods
- Tooth Rescue (emergencies — mainly for permanent teeth)
- Tough Teeth (fluorides)
- Be Cool
- Seal Out Trouble

Dental Health Foundation, 4340 Redwood Highway, Suite 319, San Rafael, CA 94903; (415) 499-4648

"Preventing Baby Bottle Tooth Decay: A Professional's Guide" (video) (target audience is caregivers)

"Protect Your Child's Teeth: Put Your Baby to Bed with Love, Not a Bottle" (easy-to-read pamphlet for parents in English, Spanish, Chinese, Cambodian, Laotian, Thai and Vietnamese)

JMH Communications, 1133 Broadway, Suite 1123, New York, NY 10010; 1-800-334-7734

> "Bright Smiles, Bright Futures" (multicultural oral health activity kit for early childhood programs; contains video, audiotape, books, parent brochures, teachers' guide, and other materials)

State Departments of Health; Office of Dental Health (available on loan)

> "Jody Says, Love Your Teeth" (teaching module for hearing-impaired preschoolers and other special needs children; includes 15-minute video, teacher's workbook, puzzles, hand puppets, and storybooks). Some states have Spanish version. Not available for purchase. For more information, contact Arizona Department of Health Services, Office of Oral Health, 1740 West Adams, Room 010, Phoenix, AZ 85007; (602) 542-1866.

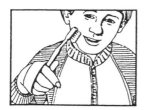

Attach brush to child's hand with wide elastic band.

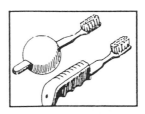

For children with limited grasp, enlarge brush handle with sponge, rubber ball, or bicycle handle grip.

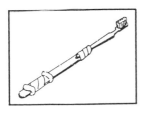

For children who can't raise their hand or arm, lengthen brush handle with ruler, tongue depressor, or long wooden spoon.

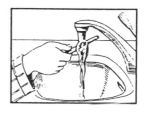

Bend brush handle by running hot water over handle (not head) of brush.

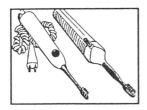

For children who can't manipulate a regular toothbrush, an electric tooth-brush may enable them to brush.

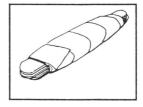

If child can't keep mouth open, use mouth prop — for example, three or four tongue depresssors taped together, a rolled-up moistened washcloth, or a rubber doorstop.[1]

Figure 1
Adapting a toothbrush
©Johnson & Johnson Consumer Products, Inc. 1989. Used by permission.

---

[1] Ask a dental professional how to use a mouth prop to avoid injuring the child's mouth.

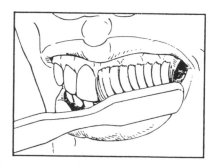 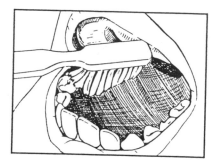

Place toothbrush bristles at the gum line, at 45-degree angle to gums. Press gently and use short strokes with back and forth, or light scrubbing motion.

Start with upper teeth, brushing outside, inside, and chewing surfaces. Do the same for lower teeth. Be sure to brush each tooth.

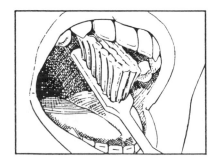 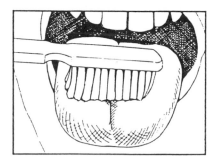

Reposition brush vertically to clean inside surfaces of front teeth, upper and lower.

To freshen breath, brush tongue, too, as tongue can harbor many bacteria

Figure 2
Step-by-step brushing
©Johnson & Johnson Consumer Products, Inc. 1989. Used by permission.

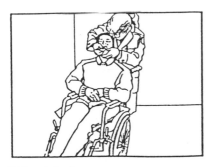

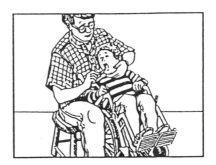

Wheelchair

Stand behind wheelchair. Use your arm to brace child's head against chair or your body. Use pillow for your child's comfort.

Or sit behind wheelchair. Remember to lock chair wheels first, then tilt chair back into your lap.

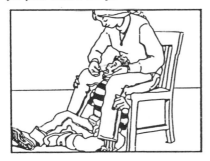

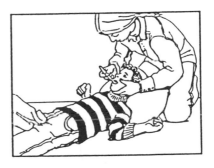

Sitting on Floor

Child sits on floor; you sit behind child's chair. Child leans head against your knees. If child is uncooperative or uncontrollable, you can place your legs over child's arms to keep child still.

Lying on floor

Child lies on floor with head on pillow. You kneel behind child's head. You can use your arm to hold child still.

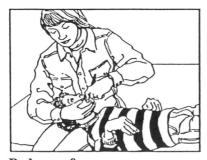

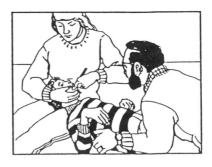

Bed or sofa

Child lies on bed or sofa with head in your lap. Support child's head and shoulders with your arm.

If child is uncooperative or uncontrollable, a second person can hold hands or feet if needed.

continued

Figure 3
Helpful positions for teeth care

Figure 3 (con't.)

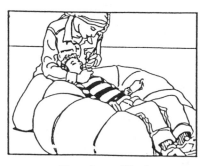

Beanbag Chair
For children who have difficulty sitting up straight, a beanbag chair lets them relax without the fear of falling. Use same position as for bed or sofa.

Figure 3 (con't.)
Helpful positions for teeth care
©Johnson & Johnson Consumer Products, Inc. 1989. Used by permission.

FIRST AID FOR COMMON CHILD CARE INCIDENTS

I. **Need**

    A. Child caregivers need to be able to handle a wide spectrum of child injuries ranging from minor to life-threatening.

    B. Child caregivers have to know how to follow specific procedures for specific conditions.

II. **First aid readiness**

    A. Caregiver preparedness

        1. Current certification in CPR is essential.

        2. Hands-on training in pediatric first aid, such as that provided by the Red Cross, is strongly recommended.

        3. Decisions

            a. All serious injuries require *immediate* contact with the Emergency Medical System (EMS). The severity of an injury is a judgment based upon training and common sense.

            b. When the injury is more than a slight cut or scratch, the caregiver should answer the following questions before calling the parent/guardian:

                (1) Does the child's behavior indicate a serious problem (considering that children have a wide range of pain tolerance)?

                (2) How understanding is the parent/guardian's employer about non-life threatening emergencies?

                (3) How much contact does the parent/guardian want? Parents of children with chronic conditions and disabilities may wish to be notified immediately of even minor incidents.

c.   If the severity of injury is in question, the parent/guardian should be called to make the decision.

d.   Notifying parents/guardians

(1)   The caregiver should carry emergency contact information at all times.

(2)   If the injury is serious, the parent/guardian should be called *after* EMS arrives (or after EMS is called if someone is available to attend to the child while awaiting EMS).

B.   Center preparedness

1.   A file for each child should contain the following:

a.   Emergency contact information including phone numbers for

(1)   parents/guardians;
(2)   alternative emergency contacts;
(3)   the child's health care provider: name, address, and phone number; and
(4)   IFSP or IEP, if applicable.

b.   Parental/guardian permission forms for emergency transportation.

2.   Child care centers should maintain sturdy listings (posted by the phone) of:

a.   the center's address and phone number (to inform emergency medical services, or EMS, as well as other emergency contacts);

b.   emergency phone numbers (including EMS, 911, local hospital emergency room, local physicians, poison control, police, fire, and so on); and

c.   the center's emergency procedures.

3.   First aid supplies

    a.   First aid kit

        (1)   Every center should keep a well stocked first aid kit, stored out of children's reach.

        (2)   The kit should include

            (a)   adhesive bandage strips (such as Band Aids™);
            (b)   gauze pads, sterile (3" x 3" and 4" x 4"), half dozen each size;
            (c)   rolled bandages (2" and 3");
            (d)   adhesive tape;
            (e)   triangle bandage (sling);
            (f)   splints (or items that may be used as splints such as tongue depressors, small/flat boards);
            (g)   scissors;
            (h)   safety pins;
            (i)   tweezers;
            (j)   bulb syringe (for cleaning eyes);
            (k)   waterless cleansing pads in sealed packets;
            (l)   book of matches (for sterilizing metal implements);
            (m)   cold packs;
            (n)   hot water bottle;
            (o)   flashlight and extra batteries;
            (p)   disposable latex gloves;
            (q)   syrup of ipecac (check expiration date);[1]
            (r)   soap; and
            (s)   pen/pencil and note pad.

        (3)   Ointments, creams, peroxide, and other over-the-counter medications commonly used at home should *not* be included in the center's first aid kit.

---

[1] Administer only if directed to do so by the Poison Control Center, following their instructions precisely.

4.   It is important to be able to get

a.   blankets, and
b.   water.

5.   You can make do with

a.   magazines used as splints, and
b.   bags of frozen peas wrapped in a cloth (to protect the skin) used as cold packs.

III.   Emergency situations

A.   A child loses consciousness.

B.   A child has a seizure.

C.   A child stops breathing.

D.   A child has *severe* bleeding, for any reason.

IV.   Emergency actions.   *The list below notes some actions that require you to be CPR-certified.*

A.   Stay calm.

B.   First steps

1.   Evaluate the scene.

a.   Can you approach the victim(s) safely?
b.   What happened?
c.   Can you account for all the children in your care?

2.   If possible, have the oldest or most responsible child gather the other children nearby you.

3.   Call over any adult bystanders to help.

C.   Assess the condition of the injured child(ren). *A problem in any of the following areas requires CPR or emergency first aid training, as well as a call for emergency medical help — EMS, a local hospital emergency room, or local physician.*

1.   Is the child conscious and responsive?

       a.   Ask, "Are you okay?" or gently tap or shake a baby's or child's shoulder.

       b.   If the child is not face up, do a log roll of the unconscious child. *Demonstrated by the instructor.*

2.   Breathing and circulation (*Certification courses are required to intervene in breathing and circulation problems competently.*)

       a.   A child who is not breathing is at risk for brain damage because the brain is not getting oxygen.

       b.   An ABC check consists of:

            (1)   *A*irway: Position the head (as taught in CPR training) so the airway is not blocked. The tongue is the most frequent obstruction. (If a head or neck injury is suspected, the airway should be cleared using the jaw-thrust method taught as part of CPR training.)

            (2)   *B*reathing: Check for breathing.

            (3)   *C*irculation: Check for a pulse and severe bleeding.

                (a)   For infants, check the brachial artery, located between the elbow and shoulder or the inner arm.

                (b)   For children, check the carotid artery, located in the groove between the windpipe and muscles at the side of the neck.

Taking pulse at side of neck

c.   To restart breathing and circulation, use *cardiopulmonary resuscitation (CPR) as taught in a CPR certification class*. Response to an ABC problem requires

(1)   positioning the head to clear the airway;
(2)   doing rescue breathing if there is a pulse but no breathing;[2] or
(3)   doing rescue breathing combined with chest compressions if there is neither pulse nor breathing.

d.   If proper positioning and repeated attempts to clear the airway are not effective, the airway may be blocked by swelling.

D.   If no ABC problems are found, check for symptoms of shock. Report problems in an EMS call.

1.   Observe breathing. Is it fast, shallow, or irregular?
2.   Feel pulse in neck or upper arm. Fast? Hard to find?
3.   Check skin appearance, moisture, and temperature.
4.   Check head for cuts, swelling, and bruises.
5.   Check ears, nose and mouth for bleeding or other discharge.
6.   Check pupils of both eyes. Enlarged? Tiny? Same size?

E.   *When an EMS or 911 call must be made*:

1.   Call EMS, 911, other local emergency service, or hospital (or emergency physician's) number posted on or by phone.

a.   Ask a responsible child to bring the phone and first aid kit to you, if possible.
b.   Ask a responsible child to get adult help, and have a responsible person stand outside to wait for the ambulance, if possible.
c.   If no other responsible person is available to call EMS, perform rescue breathing or CPR for one minute before calling.

---

[2]   Children with tracheostomies require rescue breathing through the trach tube rather than the nose and mouth.

2. Tell EMS:

   a. *Who and where* you are — your name and the center's address and phone number (address and phone number should be posted by the phone).
   b. *What* happened.
   c. *How many* victims and their condition.
   d. *First aid* being given.

3. Stay on the line until EMS hangs up to make sure you have answered all questions.

4. Keep the children in your care nearby you if no other adult is present.

5. Do not try to transport the child to the hospital yourself (except in cases of natural disasters or other unusual circumstances).

F. After an EMS call, follow instructions received in the call.

G. Comfort and reassure the child(ren).

V. Most common injuries in child care

A. Cuts and scrapes

B. Human bites

C. Eye injuries

D. Poisoning

E. Exposure injuries (such as burns from hot slides and overexposure to cold)

F. See Table 1 for severity levels of common child care injuries.

Table 1
Severity of common child care emergencies

Condition	Minor	Serious	Life-threatening
Bites/stings			
insect, nonpoisonous	X		
insect, with generalized swelling		X	
insect, with breathing difficulty			X
human bite	X		
human bite, with broken skin	X	X	
animal, with broken skin		X	
animal, with excessive bleeding			X
Cuts/wounds			
scrape/scratch	X		
with some bleeding	X		
with difficult-to-control bleeding		X	
with spurting blood loss			X
Burns: thermal or chemical[3]	X	X	X
sunburn	X	X	
bleach spilled on genitals			X
Water accidents			
taking in a mouth & nose full of water	X		
head injury while diving			X

continued

---

[3] Burns differ in severity from mild to life threatening. See following discussion in Care of Common Injuries.

Table 1 (con't.)

Condition	Minor	Serious	Life-threatening
Foreign objects/substances			
object in ear		X	
sand in eye	X	X	
chemical in eye		X	
object in nose	X		
object or food lodged in throat			X
Falls			
swollen ankle	X		
inability to move fingers/toes		X	
bone piercing skin		X	
Weather-related conditions			
frostbite		X	
heat exhaustion		X	
heat stroke			X
Head injuries			
bump on head with some swelling	X		
blow to head with drowsiness/vomiting		X	
blow to head with fluid seeping from ears			X
fractured skull			X
Poisoning			
toddler swallows dish detergent	X		
toddler swallows liquid antibiotic		X	

continued

Table 1 (con't.)

Condition	*Minor*	*Serious*	*Life-threatening*
Injury to teeth			
cracked		X	
broken		X	
Nosebleeds	X		
Shock			X

VI. Care of common injuries

   A.   Bites

      1.   Human bites

         a.   Wash the wound with soap and water.
         b.   If the skin is broken, apply sterile dressing.
         c.   Tell the parent/guardian that medical care will be required if the wound becomes infected. Some physicians recommend treatment with antibiotics in all cases if the skin is broken.

      2.   Insect bites and stings

         a.   Do not mash the insect; save it for identification.
         b.   Remove stinger only if it is sticking out and removed easily by scraping it (with a credit card, for example); don't use tweezers or fingernails.
         c.   Wash the wound with soap and water.
         d.   Apply a cold pack.
         e.   Call EMS if a severe reaction occurs (signaled by paleness, difficulty breathing, rapid and weak pulse, sickness).

   B.   Bleeding (from wounds, cuts, and scrapes)

      1.   *Use gloves* (at all times during child care, keep latex gloves readily available, in pocket or waist pack).

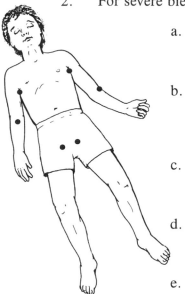

Pressure points

2.   For severe bleeding:

a.   *Cover the wound* with a dressing (preferably sterile gauze, but don't waste time).

b.   *Apply direct pressure* and *elevate the wound* (unless a fracture is suspected), adding more pads on top of blood-soaked gauze.

c.   Keep the wound elevated, maintain direct pressure, and *press on pressure points*.

d.   *Apply a pressure bandage*, tying the knot directly over the gauze pads.

e.   *Treat for shock* while waiting for EMS to arrive.

3.   For cuts and scrapes:

a.   Abrasions (skin is scraped but little or no bleeding)

(1)   Clean area of scrape with soap and water.
(2)   May cover with Band Aid™ or bandage.

b.   Minor cuts (only a small amount of bleeding)

(1)   Clean area with soap and water and blot dry.
(2)   Apply dry, sterile bandage (dressing).

4.   To remove blood-contaminated gloves:

a.   Grasp the glove at the palm side of the wrist, rolling/pulling so the glove turns inside as you slip it off.

b.   Dispose of used gloves, bloody tissues, bandages, and other bloodied items in a plastic bag and secure it.

c.   Wash hands thoroughly.

C.   Burns

    1.   Severity is determined by

        a.   degree (amount of tissue damage);
        b.   size;
        c.   location on body (critical areas are hands, face, feet, genitals);
        d.   child's age (most critical on infants, toddlers); and
        e.   presence of any disability in which the child does not feel pain.

    2.   Types and symptoms

        a.   First degree: Red skin, mild swelling, pain
        b.   Second degree: Red skin, blistering (open or closed), severe pain
        c.   Third degree: Red, white, or charred skin; loss of skin layers. May or may not be painful. Skin grafts required.

    3.   Burns that need immediate medical care

        a.   Smoke or flame inhalation in addition to burn
        b.   Burn in which the child can not be comforted
        c.   Blistering burn larger than a bottle cap on a very young child
        d.   Third degree burn of any size
        e.   Burn on a child with a chronic health problem
        f.   Burn on critical areas of the body
        g.   Injuries in addition to burn
        h.   Burn that may indicate abuse

    4.   When clothes catch on fire, follow the maxim: *stop, drop, and roll.*

    5.   Actions for heat burns

        a.   *Check ABCs* (see section IV. Emergency actions).
        b.   Call EMS as needed.
        c.   Use *water* to cool all burns of limited size. Flush with or submerge in cool (*not iced*) water. *Do not* apply sprays, ointments or other remedies. For third degree burns over large areas, cover with a clean dry wrap to prevent hypothermia.

      d.   Remove clothing around the burn, *unless* stuck to burned area. If stuck, *do not attempt to remove.*

      e.   Apply a dry, sterile dressing *loosely.*

      f.   Treat for shock as needed.

6.   Chemical burns

      a.   *Call EMS.*

      b.   Flush chemicals off with running water for 15 to 30 minutes. If a lot of water is not available, brush chemical off the skin. The child's eyes should be closed or protected from the dust.

      c.   Cover area(s) loosely with a dry dressing,

7.   Electrical burns

      a.   *Stay away from live current* to avoid being shocked yourself.

          (1)   In emergencies outdoors, *do not touch downed power lines.* Call the power company.

          (2)   In emergencies indoors, *shut off the power* (at the circuit breaker or fuse box).

      b.   Be aware that the victim may experience cardiac arrest (the heart stops beating).

      c.   *Call EMS.*

      d.   Cover burn(s) loosely with a dry dressing.

      e.   Treat for shock.

8.   Sunburn

      a.   Prevent sunburn by limiting exposure to the sun, both time spent in the sun and proper attire (such as hats and light fabrics to cover the skin).

      b.   Use sunscreen in accordance with center policy (which should require parental permission and parental provision of the product).

D.   Drowning

1.   Throw a towel, life preserver, branch, or other item to keep the child afloat and to pull him/her toward you.

2.   If a head, neck, or back injury is suspected, do not jerk or twist the body while removing the child from the water.

3.   *Monitor ABCs (section IV). Perform rescue breathing or CPR as needed.*

4.   If the child vomits, log roll onto side (moving head, neck, and back as one unit).

5.   Inform the parent/guardian even if the incident seems minor; fluid in the lungs can cause pneumonia.

E.   Ear: foreign object in ear

1.   Turn head, with obstructed (blocked) side down.

2.   *Do not attempt to remove the object.* You could push it farther into the ear.

3.   Call parent/guardian to seek medical care immediately.

F.   Eye injuries

1.   Foreign object (such as an eyelash or sand) in eye

a.   Wash your hands and the child's hands.
b.   Remove debris from *lower lid* with slightly damp, clean cloth. Do not use tissue or cotton.
c.   Remove debris from *upper lid* by pulling the lid out, down, and then upward, folding lid back while the child looks down.
d.   Rinse the eye with water, flowing in the direction from the nose toward the ear.

2.   Chemicals in eye

a.   *Call EMS.*
b.   If struggling inhibits rinsing, wrap the child's arms and legs in large towel.
c.   Encourage the child to blink frequently; do not use excessive force to open the eye.
d.   Flush the eye with lots of water, flowing in the direction from the nose toward the ear.

3.   Lacerated (cut) eyeball or object impaled into eyeball

a.   *Call EMS.*

     b.   *Do not remove* an impaled object.

     c.   *Do not wash or apply pressure.*

     d.   Cover both eyes with a loose bandage.

     e.   Treat for shock while waiting for EMS to arrive.

G.   Fractures, dislocations, strains, sprains

    1.   Symptoms of fractures

        a.   Pain

        b.   Swelling, bruising

        c.   Inability to move fingers/toes

        d.   Deformity, a body part appears different from its mate on the opposite side

    2.   Actions

        a.   If bone has broken through the skin:

           (1)   *Call EMS.*

           (2)   Stop bleeding (use pressure point rather than direct pressure).

        b.   Immobilize limbs *without straightening or bending them.*

        c.   Use pillows, jackets, blankets to elevate and immobilize the injury.

        d.   *Do not* use stretch ("Ace") bandages.

        e.   For foot/ankle injuries, remove or loosen the shoe if it can be done without moving or jarring the injured area.

        f.   Apply cold packs on both sides of the injury.

        g.   Treat dislocations, strains, and sprains like a fracture.

H.   Frostbite

    1.   Symptoms

        a.   White or yellow color to nose, ears, cheeks, fingers, toes, and affected parts feel hard

        b.   Pain changing to numbness as frostbite worsens

        c.   Possible blistering

    2.   Actions

        a.   Bring the child indoors.

        b.   *Do not rub or massage.*

    c.   Cover the child gently with blankets.

    d.   Remove blankets when frozen areas looked flushed.

    e.   Give the child a warm drink, but never alcohol.

    f.   If toes or fingers are affected, separate with gauze, then bandage loosely.

    g.   Seek medical care immediately.

I.   Head, neck, and back injuries

    1.   Serious injuries

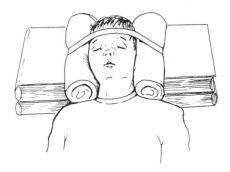

Immobilization of head

    a.   *Do not attempt to move* the child (except in extreme danger of further injury). If possible, prevent movement by placing rolled blankets, towel, and the like by the sides of the child's head. Pack heavy items (for example, books) around the outer edges of the blankets to keep them in place.

    b.   *Check ABCs* (see section IV. Emergency actions).

    c.   *Call EMS.*

    d.   If bleeding from nose or mouth:

        (1)   Log roll (move head, neck, and back as one unit) onto side.

        (2)   Do not attempt to stop blood flow.

        (3)   Maintain ABCs while waiting for EMS.

    2.   Minor head injuries

    a.   Apply cold compress.

    b.   Observe the child closely for signs of drowsiness, shock, or vomiting. Vomiting may occur once as a normal response to the stress of the accident. If it continues, it is not normal.

    c.   Require the child to rest before resuming normal activity.

    d.   If you've been instructed to check for consciousness, interrupt the child's sleep after 20 minutes.

J.   Heat stroke

    1.   Symptoms

      a.   Hot, dry, red skin (the child has stopped sweating)

      b.   Strong, rapid pulse

      c.   Possible unconsciousness

  2.   Actions

      a.   *Call EMS.*

      b.   Move the child to shade.

      c.   Remove the child's clothing.

      d.   Sponge with cool water, starting with the head.

      e.   Fan the face and body.

      f.   *Do not* give an unconscious child anything to drink. If the child is alert, give small sips of cool water.

      g.   Care for shock.

K.   Heat exhaustion

  1.   Symptoms

      a.   Pale, clammy skin

      b.   Profuse sweating

      c.   Weakness, dizziness

      d.   Nausea, vomiting

      e.   Pupils of eyes dilated (expanded)

  2.   Actions

      a.   Move the child to shade.

      b.   Loosen the child's clothing.

      c.   Apply cool, wet cloths.

      d.   Give sips of water if the child is not vomiting.

L.   Mouth injuries

  1.   Cracked tooth (whole tooth is still intact)

      a.   Place a cold pack on the child's face next to the broken tooth.

      b.   Call the parent/guardian and advise prompt care by dentist.

  2.   Tooth knocked out or broken

      a.   Place the tooth in a glass of milk (if available), water, or moist gauze.

      b.   *Do not* attempt to wash or clean the tooth.

        c.   Call the parent/guardian to take the child to a dentist immediately.

    3.   Tongue/lips bleeding

        a.   Use gloves (and universal precautions for removal and disposal when through with them).
        b.   Cover the wound with gauze and apply direct pressure.

M.   Nosebleeds (minor)

    1.   Use gloves (and universal precautions for removing and disposing when through with them).
    2.   Keep the child in a sitting position with the head forward.
    3.   Pinch the child's nose for 2 - 5 minutes to allow blood to clot.
    4.   Keep the child quiet for 5 - 10 minutes.
    5.   Keep the child from blowing the nose for 1 hour or more.

N.   Nose: foreign object in nose

    1.   Encourage the child to breathe through the mouth.
    2.   Ask the child to blow the nose gently, keeping both nostrils open.
    3.   If the object does not come out, or if the child is too young to blow on command, seek medical care immediately.

O.   Poisoning

    1.   *Call Poison Control, EMS, or a local emergency room or physician's office immediately.*

        a.   Do not administer treatment before talking with Poison Control. This includes antidote directions on the poison's container.

        b.   *Take the poison's container and the child's medical records to the phone.* Be prepared to answer:

            (1)   How many victims?
            (2)   What was taken?
            (3)   How was it taken (inhaled, spilled on skin, swallowed)?
            (4)   How much was taken?

(5) If the amount is unknown, assume that the child has taken the entire amount missing.

(6) How much does the child weigh? (Weights of all children should be checked periodically, dated and documented in health records.) Dosages of antidotes are based on body weight.

(7) Does the child have any allergies or other health problems?

2. Inhaled fumes:

   a. Take the child outside or away from the contaminated area.
   b. Ventilate the room.
   c. Begin rescue breathing if needed.

3. Poison on skin

   a. *See* Burns, chemical, page 277.
   b. For poison ivy and the like:
      (1) remove the child's clothing, and
      (2) wash skin with soap and water.

4. Poison in eyes

   a. *See* Eye injuries, chemical, page 278.
   b. *Call Poison Control.*

P. Seizures

1. Signs of a seizure may include any or none of the following:

   a. An aura, a specific sensation (a smell, memory, feeling, or sound), the child recognizes as a warning sign;
   b. A prodrome, a feeling of fear or anxiety that occurs days or hours before a seizure, causing young children to seek out a parent or caregiver and to look apprehensive;
   c. the eyes rolling back or moving to one side or the other, or moving jerkily;
   d. regular, rhythmic patterns of muscle movement in all or part of the body, including jerking or twitching, or a repetitive activity such as blinking, chewing, or picking at something;

e.   impairment or loss of consciousness, or unresponsiveness; and/or

f.   pallor of the face or a bluish color around the lips and/or nail beds.

2.   When you notice the signs:

a.   In a safe place where you can closely observe him/her, turn the child (or child's head) to side.

b.   If child has vomited, try to clean out the mouth and nose to prevent choking.

c.   Do not try to pry the child's mouth open or put anything in his/her mouth.

d.   Remove hard objects from thrashing range, but do not restrain the arms or legs.

e.   Place a blanket or pillow under the child's head.

f.   Remove tight, restrictive clothing from around the neck.

g.   Stay with the child throughout the seizure, comforting and keeping him/her calm and quiet.

h.   Do not give food, drink, or a bottle until the child is fully awake.

i.   Time the episode with a watch.

3.   An emergency situation exists if

a.   the seizure lasts more than 20 minutes, or

b.   the child has continuous seizures, or

c.   the child remains unconscious after the seizure, or

d.   he/she stops breathing.

4.   Contact emergency medical assistance, start CPR if appropriate, and contact the child's parent/guardian.

Q.   *Shock* results from inadequate blood flow to the brain, heart, lungs, and other vital organs. First aid for shock should be performed for all serious injuries as soon as the primary problem (breathing, bleeding, and so on) is under control.

1.   Symptoms

a.   Very fast, weak pulse

b.   Irregular breathing

c.   Trembling and weakness

    d.   Moist, clammy skin

    e.   Nausea, dizziness

2.   Actions

    a.   Positioning the victim

        (1)   Standard shock position and position for unknown injuries

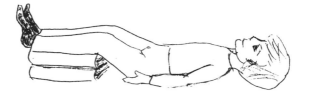

Standard shock position

        (2)   Position for suspected spinal injury

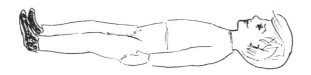

Shock position for suspected head and neck injury

        (3)   Position for head injuries/breathing difficulties

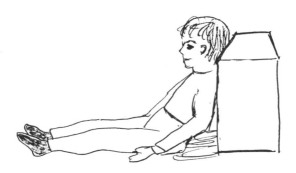

Shock position for breathing difficulties

(4)   Position for vomiting, bleeding from mouth

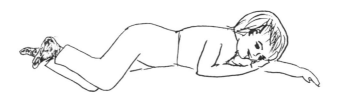

Shock position for vomiting

b.   Temperature control

(1)   To keep the child from chilling, place one blanket under the child if it is safe to do so. (If the child has an unknown injury, or a spinal injury, *do not* move the child more than is necessary to open the airway.)

(2)   Monitor the child for overheating.

c.   Do not give the child anything to drink.

VII. Follow-up

A.   Complete the documentation for incident or accident reports as required by your center. While still fresh in your mind:

1.   Record names, addresses, phone numbers of witnesses, bystanders, or other adults who helped during the incident.

2.   State where other staff members were at the time of the incident.

3.   Describe your response and how much time went by before help arrived.

B.   Restock the first aid kit.

VIII. Implications for children with special needs

A.   Examples of physical disabilities and conditions

1.   Shift the position of a child in a wheelchair, braces, or other adaptive equipment periodically (as taught)

to prevent pressure sores. The child may not feel the pain of a developing sore.

2. Be aware that inactivity reduces circulation to extremities. Children with limited mobility are more at risk for hypothermia and frostbite. Some children may not feel pain from freezing tissues.

3. Take special care with adaptive equipment such as oxygen therapy apparatus and home cardiac/ respiratory monitors that have electrical wires or long tubing. Electric shock, tripping over wires or tubing, or disconnecting the child accidentally from the apparatus are possible risks.

4. With children who have visual or auditory impairments, ensure a safe environment (free of potentially harmful objects and substances) and be able to communicate in threatening situations.

5. Be aware of the triggers of asthma attacks (for example, cold weather) and of signs of respiratory distress.

6. For children with seizure disorders, be alert to early warning signs (if known) of an impending seizure to minimize injuries from possible falls.

B. Cognitive disabilities

1. When dealing with children who have cognitive disabilities and developmental delays, adjust your expectations concerning their memories for safety rules and the like.

2. Be aware of limits on the activities of children with some cognitive disabilities (such as Down syndrome) who have a tendency to fall and dislocate joints.

BIBLIOGRAPHY

American Red Cross (1988). *American Red Cross standard first aid: Workbook*.

American Red Cross (1990). *American Red Cross child care course: health and safety units: Workbook*.

Eberlein, T. (1993). This is only a test...But it could help you do the right thing in case of emergency. See how much you know about first aid. *American Baby: For Expectant and New Parents, 55(10)*, 36, 38, 40.

Green, M. (1989). *A sigh of relief (3d ed.)*. West Stockbridge, MA: Berkshire Studio.

National Safety Council (1993). *First aid and CPR: Infants and children*. Boston: Jones and Bartlett.

Vogel, S., & Manhoff, D. (1984). *Emergency medical treatment: Children*. Wilmette, IL: EMT Inc. in cooperation with National Safety Council.

RESOURCES

American Red Cross, National Headquarters Health and Safety, 18th & F Streets, N.W., Washington, D.C. 20006; (202) 737-8300

American Heart Association, 7272 Greenville Avenue, Dallas, TX 75231; (214) 373-6300

National Child Safety Council, 4065 Page Avenue, P.O. Box 1368, Jackson, MI 49204; (517) 764-6070

ENVIRONMENTAL SAFETY

I. **Safety principles**

    A. Children have a natural curiosity that stimulates exploration of their environment and learning but *also* may place them in jeopardy of falling, ingesting hazardous objects, and so forth.

    B. Safety measures apply to children at different developmental stages rather than at different age levels.

    C. Some children may be delayed motorically in some way but not delayed cognitively; others may be delayed cognitively but not motorically; and so on.

    D. Providing a controlled and safe environment is the responsibility of caregivers.

        1. Caregivers should be sensitive to under- and over-dressing children for the building temperature.

        2. Caregivers should keep children with balance problems away from sharp objects and areas with hard floors.

        3. Caregivers should look at the environment from the child's perspective — on hands and knees.

II. **Accidents**

    A. Accidents are the leading cause of death of children at all ages.

    B. Common types of accidents that cause death in children

        1. Auto collisions

            a. Auto accidents are a leading cause of death among children.
            b. Many permanent injuries also occur.
            c. Prevention.

                (1) Use seat restraints (largely mandated by state law).
                (2) Use safety seats for all children (largely mandated by state law).

       (3)   Teach street safety to children who are able to understand it.

       (4)   Do not allow children to play near high-traffic areas.

2.   Falls

    a.   Children can fall out of windows, down stairs, off beds/changing tables, and from playground equipment.

    b.   Most injuries in the child care setting occur on the playground.

    c.   Prevention.

       (1)   Never leave an infant unattended on a changing table or a bed or an infant seat that is not on the floor.

       (2)   Use gates at top and bottom of stairs.

       (3)   Secure all window screens.

       (4)   Remove furniture with sharp edges or pad it effectively.

       (5)   Keep crib rails raised.

       (6)   Use restraint (built-in) in highchairs.

       (7)   Keep shoelaces tied.

       (8)   On the playground:

          (a)   Inspect playground equipment regularly for sharp edges, wood splinters, broken or weakened parts.

          (b)   Supervise children's play continuously, especially in getting down and climbing up equipment. Older children tend to prod younger children to go beyond their limits.

3.   Choking/suffocation

    a.   Toys and food cause most choking accidents.

    b.   Prevention.

       (1)   Do not have toys with small, removable parts.

       (2)   Be watchful for stray buttons, beads, and other small objects, and remove them from the area.

(3)   In children under 3 years old, avoid

  (a)   peanuts,
  (b)   popcorn,
  (c)   hot dogs, and
  (d)   hard candy.

(4)   Do not feed infants when they are lying down.
(5)   Do not use balloons as toys.
(6)   Know emergency measures including

  (a)   back slaps,
  (b)   Heimlich maneuver, and
  (c)   when to call 911.

(7)   Do not use soft, large pillows, especially around infants who have difficulty with head control.

4.   Smoke inhalation, fires and burns, and secondhand smoke

  a.   Fires kill or injure thousands of children every year.
  b.   Prevention.

  (1)   Know and adhere to state licensing requirements regarding

    (a)   smoke detectors,
    (b)   escape routes, and
    (c)   fire extinguishers.

  (2)   Keep matches away from children (toddlers are most at-risk).
  (3)   Be aware that young children have thinner, more sensitive skin than adults and are burned more easily by hot water, coffee, and so forth.
  (4)   Keep hot water heater temperature between 100° F. and 125° F.
  (5)   Avoid overexposing children to sun.
  (6)   Check food temperatures before offering food to children.
  (7)   Cover electrical outlets.

        (8)   Encourage parents/guardians to clothe infants in fire-retardant pajamas and other clothing.

        (9)   Do not expose children to secondhand smoke.

5.   Poisoning

    a.   Poisoning is a major cause of death in children younger than 5 years old.

    b.   Poisonings happen most often in settings that are not "child-proofed," such as grandparents' or friends' houses.

    c.   Prevention.

        (1)   Keep all medications in a locked cabinet or cupboard.

        (2)   Always use safety caps on medicines.

        (3)   Keep medicines in their original containers.

        (4)   Lock cupboards containing cleaning supplies and dangerous substances.

        (5)   Never call medicine "candy."

        (6)   Remove poisonous plants (several common house plants are poisonous).

    d.   Keep local/regional poison control center numbers visible on or next to the phone.

6.   Drowning

    a.   Individuals cannot live long without oxygen, so adults must act quickly to save children from drowning.

    b.   Prevention.

        (1)   Although young children may be able to sit well and walk, never leave them alone in a bathtub. Bathtubs are slippery, and if a child falls in the water, even one inch, he/she may not be able to sit up again and can drown.

        (2)   Take the same precautions with wading pools.

III. Accident prevention associated with developmental milestones

A. Gross-motor

1. Involuntary reflexes (0-4 months)

   a. Do not leave an infant alone on the changing table or any raised surface that does not have guards.
   b. Keep plastic bags away from infants.
   c. Do not use plastic to cover pillows or mattresses.
   d. Do not tie a pacifier around an infant's neck.
   e. Keep crib rails raised.
   f. Always use an approved car seat.
   g. Do not put diaper pins and other sharp objects on the changing table.

2. Rolling over (2-5 months)

   a. Keep small objects and toy parts out of reach of infants.
   b. Restrain infants properly in highchairs.
   c. Lock up cleaning supplies and medicines.
   d. Keep plants out of the reach of infants.
   e. Keep hot objects and liquids out of reach.
   f. Keep at least one hand on the child on the changing table if you have to turn away.

3. Mouthing reflex (4-7 months)

   a. Do not have toys with sharp or small parts, such as stuffed animals with plastic eyes.
   b. Keep diaper pins closed and away from infants.
   c. Do not use balloons as toys, as they can cause suffocation.
   d. Do not feed an infant hard candy, nuts, foods with pits or seeds, or whole hot dogs.

4. Crawling (7-10 months)

   a. Use gates at the top and bottom of stairs.
   b. Supervise children in and around any water.
   c. Keep large appliance doors closed.
   d. Do not call medicine "candy."
   e. Use safety caps on medicine.
   f. Put safety guards over electric outlets.

5.   Standing/walking (6-14 months)

      a.   Avoid dangling tablecloths that the child can pull.

      b.   Be sure outside play areas are well fenced.

      c.   Use sturdy car restraints as required by law.

      d.   Lock gates and doors.

      e.   Turn pot handles toward the back of the stove.

      f.   Keep electrical appliances and tools out of reach of children.

      g.   Supervise children closely in outdoor play areas.

6.   Climbing (14-18 months)

      a.   Keep cleaning supplies locked away.

      b.   Have screens on windows.

      c.   Keep hot liquids (such as coffee) out of reach of children.

      d.   Keep sharp objects (such as scissors) away from the child's access.

7.   Pedaling tricycle or bicycle

      a.   Make sure a tricycle/bicycle is in good working order (brakes, tires) and that it is the proper size for the child.

      b.   Teach street safety.

      c.   Supervise the child continuously when outside.

      d.   Begin early with use of a safety helmet so the child is used to it as he/she grows.

B.   Fine-motor

    1.   Reaching for objects (3-5) months

      a.   Keep plastic bags away from infants.

      b.   Avoid small toys, loose buttons, hard candy, nuts, balloons, plants, hot objects, and sharp objects.

    2.   Pincer grasp (9-14 months)

      a.   Keep small toys and objects off the floor.

      b.   Keep raisins, nuts, and seeds out of the child's reach.

IV. Intellectual development (curiosity)

A. Preventive measures for caregivers

1. Encourage parents to check the neighborhood for construction sites, large holes, discarded refrigerators, and the like.

2. Encourage parents to check and be sure that neighborhood swimming pools are fenced and the gates are closed at all times.

3. Keep purses out of reach and do not allow children to play in purses that have matches, cigarettes, coins, and so on. An older child may give harmful objects to younger children.

B. Ideas for "Tip of the Week" for busy parents

1. Keep all handguns out of sight of young children. Keep gun and ammunition locked separately. Do not clean a gun in front of a child.

2. Keep household tools (saws, racks, hammers) out of reach of young children. Teach them about proper use when an adult is present.

3. Keep garden sprays and household cleaners locked up. Young children's curiosity may cause them to drink products that smell bad, just because the container looks like a "soda."

4. Teach children to care for their own pets but keep away from other animals until an adult can be present.

BIBLIOGRAPHY

Gardephe, C. D. (1994). Babyproofing: Now is the time. *American Baby: For Expectant and New Parents, 56*(10), B4, B6-9.

Holida, A. L. (1993). Latex balloons: They can take your breath away. *Pediatric Nursing, 19*(1), 39-43.

Lie, L., Runyan, C. W., Petridou, E., & Chang, A. (1994). American Public Health Association/American Academy of Pediatrics injury prevention standards. *Pediatrics, 94*(6, Pt. 2), 1046-1048.

Schneider, P. (1995). Accidents you can prevent: The six greatest dangers to your baby, and what to do right now. *Parent's Magazine, 70*(1), 56-58, 60.

Strauman-Raymond, K., Lie, L., & Kempf-Berkseth, J. (1993). Creating a safe environment for children in daycare. *Journal of School Health, 63*(6), 254-257.

Valluzzi, J. L. (1995). Safety issues in community-based setting for children who are medically fragile: Program planning for natural disasters. *Infant & Young Children, 7*(4), 62-76.

HANDLING PRINCIPLES AND TECHNIQUES

I.   **Definition of handling:** Assisting the child to move by holding or moving the child in ways that make the activity easier.

II. **Who benefits from special handling techniques?**

   A.   Special handling benefits children who have difficulty with too much or too little movement or with maintaining a position to perform an activity.

   B.   Caregivers will have more success and exert less physical effort by using specific handling techniques when working with children with special needs.

III. **Why are handling techniques important?**

   A.   Proper handling techniques reinforce the child's normal movement patterns for everyday activities such as dressing and eating.

   B.   Proper handling helps relax or improve abnormal muscle tone and reflexes.

   C.   Caregivers are less fatigued and incur fewer injuries when handling the children.

IV. **Basics of handling**

   A.   Use key points of

      1.   shoulders,

      2.   shoulder girdle,

      3.   hips, and

      4.   pelvis.

   B.   Work for symmetry.

   C.   Decrease and remove support as soon as possible.

   D.   Do not let the child overdo.

   E.   Move the child slowly.

F. Tell the child what is going to happen — what you are going to help him/her do or do to him/her such as bathing, feeding, move to another place.

G. Check with parents/guardians or child's therapist for specific techniques that work well with the child.

H. Use adaptive equipment as needed.

V. Specifics of handling

A. Feeding the child

1. Position appropriately for the child's age and ability.

2. Provide correct positioning to encourage self-feeding, (see Figures 1 - 3).

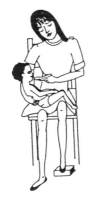
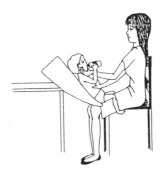

Figure 1
Semi-sitting position

Figure 2
Semi-sitting using a wedge

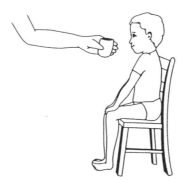

Figure 3
Correct positioning of child in chair

3. Keep the child's head centered and forward, arms forward, back rounded, hips and knees bent, and feet supported.

4. Avoid incorrect handling/positioning (Figures 4 and 5).

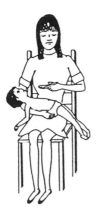 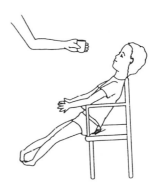

Figure 4
Incorrect position for feeding a child

Figure 5
Incorrect position for drinking from cup

B. Diapering

1. Position on back or side.

2. Bending one leg at a time lift it up and across body with knee bent. Slip diaper under that side (Figure 6).

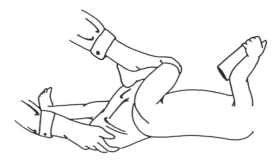

Figure 6
Diapering: first step

3. Then lift other leg the same way and slip diaper under other side (Figure 7).

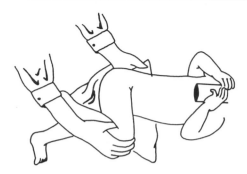

Figure 7
Diapering: second step

4. Complete the diapering, avoiding holding both legs together and pulling them straight up (Figure 8).

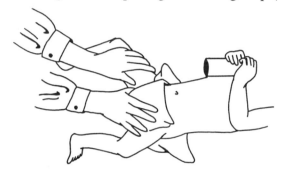

Figure 8
Diapering: final step

C. Dressing

  1. Positions

     a. Lay the child on his/her stomach over your lap.
     b. Roll from side to side to change diaper and put on clothing.
     c. Sit the child on your lap.

  2. Keeping the child's head forward, push arms through, and twist trunk to help bend legs up.

  3. Let the child help as much as possible, and talk him/her through it.

  4. To put on shoes: Bend leg at hip, knee, and ankle to make it easier to get stiff foot into shoe (Figures 9 and 10).

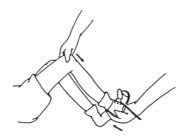

Figure 9	**Figure 10**
Putting on shoes: first step	*Putting on shoes: final step*

D. Toilet training

    1. Use the same positioning as sitting in a chair.

    2. Try elevating the knees 10°-20° above the hips.

    3. Provide something for the child to hang onto.

    4. Ask parent/guardian for specifics.

E. Bathing

    1. Put the child in a semi-sitting or sitting position.

    2. Use rolled towels or adaptive equipment.

    3. Use warm water to decrease muscle tone.

    4. Help the child to feel secure, as insecurity tightens muscles.

F. Carrying (Figures 11 - 19)

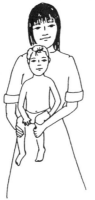

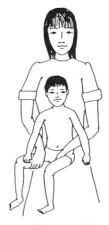

Figure 11
Carrying a child so he/she can look around

Figure 12
Carrying a stiff child

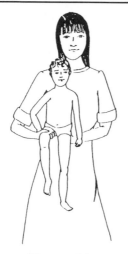

Figure 13
Carrying a child with one leg flexed

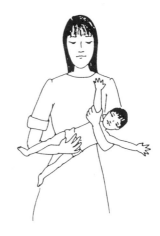

Figure 14
Side-lying is a method of carrying

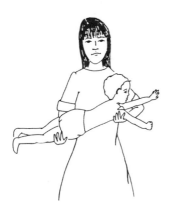

Figure 15
Carrying a child on the stomach

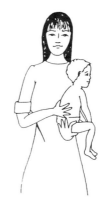

Figure 16
Carrying a floppy child

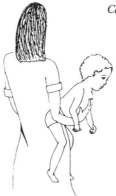

Figure 17
Carrying a stiff child

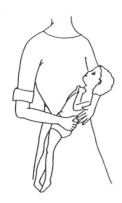

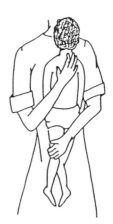

Figure 18
Incorrect way to carry a stiff child:
poor head support

Figure 19
Incorrect way to carry a stiff child:
legs straight

1. Follow the basic principles of handling or carrying the child.

2. Carry children properly to help them relax and learn better head control, as well as to make the caregiver's job easier.

3. Keep carrying to a minimum, as the child needs time to learn to move on his/her own.

4. Lifting the child: Bend your knees and lift the child using your legs, not your back.

G. Playing

1. Choose toys, games, and books that are appropriate for each child.

2. If the child is mobile, ask parent/guardian or therapist which play positions to encourage. Also ask how to discourage undesirable positions.

3. Position well, according to activity, in different positions and places
(Figures 20 - 24).

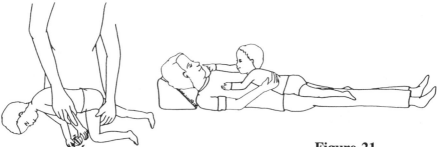

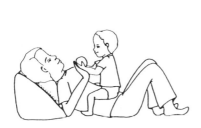

Figure 21
Laying child on his/her stomach

Figure 20
Placing child in side-lying position

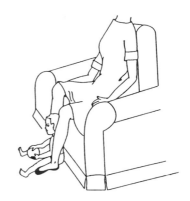

Figure 22
Playing with a child straddling your stomach

Figure 23
Using your legs and feet and a chair

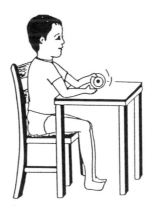

Figure 24
Correct sitting in a chair

H.   Relaxing specific problem areas of the body

    1.   Recognize abnormal postures (Figures 25 - 28).

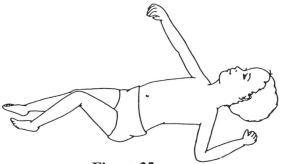

Figure 25
Typical posture of a stiff child lying on his/her back

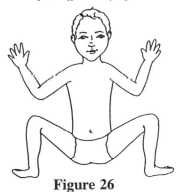

Figure 26
Typical posture of floppy child lying on his/her back

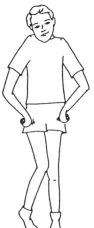

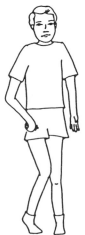

Figure 27
Typical standing posture of spastic diplegic child

Figure 28
Typical standing posture of spastic hemiplegic child

2.   Move the body part slowly until you feel resistance, then stop and wait. You will feel the body part relax. Then move slowly.

3.   Dispel the fear, as it causes muscles to tighten.

4.   Use rhythmic, repetitive movements to relax muscles.

5.   Use specific helpful techniques and avoid incorrect techniques (Figures 29 - 47).

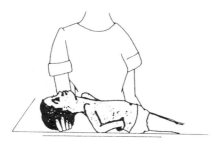

Figure 29
Incorrect handling for head pushed back

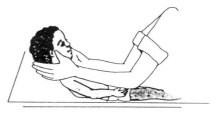

Figure 30
Correct handling for head pushed back

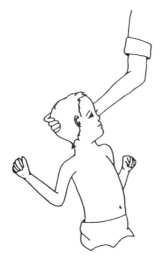

Figure 31
Incorrect assistance for arching backward

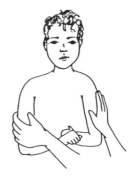

Figure 32
Correct assistance to make head come forward

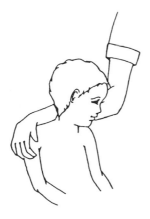

Figure 33
Holding to help head stay forward

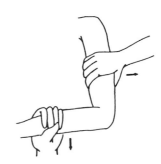

Figure 34
Incorrect way to straighten arm

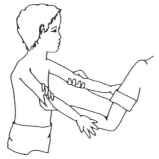

Figure 35
Correct way to straighten arm

Figure 36
Fisted hand

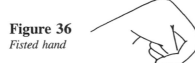

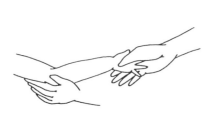

Figure 37
Opening a fisted hand: first step

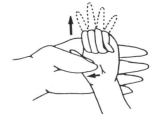

Figure 38
Opening a fisted hand: final step

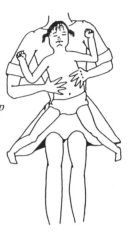

Figure 39
Incorrect: legs straddling the lap

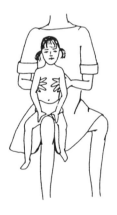

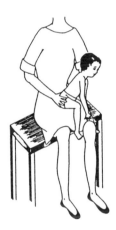

Figure 40
*Correct: sitting on one leg with
the legs comfortably apart*

Figure 41
Arms down in correct position

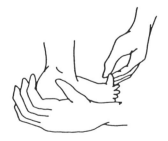

Figure 42
Relaxing toe curling

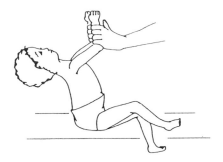

Figure 43

Incorrect: pulling a floppy or spastic child to sit

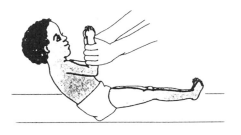

Figure 44

Incorrect: pulling a stiff child to sit

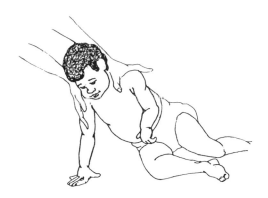

Figure 45

Correct: rotating the child while bringing him/her up to sit

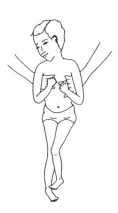

Figure 46

Incorrect: bouncing a child

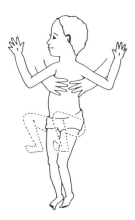

Figure 47

Incorrect: throwing a child in the air

POSITIONING AND ADAPTIVE EQUIPMENT

I. **Definition**

   A. *Positioning:* placing the child in positions in which he/she may function to the best of his/her ability.

   B. *Adaptive equipment:* any assistive device, commercial or homemade, used to maximize function and potential and minimize the child's efforts to interact with his/her environment.

II. **Who needs positioning and adaptive equipment?**

   A. Children without disabilities have variability of movement; they can move all parts of their bodies and learn to move normally through the developmental sequence.

   B. Children who have difficulty moving any part of their body need positioning to allow them a variety of movement they cannot achieve by themselves. These include children with:

      1. *Cerebral palsy:* the brain does not send the correct messages to move normally.

      2. *Spina bifida:* the spinal cord has been damaged causing some degree of paralysis.

      3. *Muscle disease:* abnormal muscle tissue makes the muscles weak.

      4. *Down syndrome (and other chromosomal abnormalities):* these children tend to be floppy or weak.

      5. *Children with other chronic illnesses* such as lung or heart disease frequently are weak, making movement difficult.

III. **Why are positioning and adaptive equipment important?**

   A. Positioning makes every activity easier for both the child and the caregiver.

   B. Each child can be helped to develop to his/her maximum potential.

   C. Appropriate positioning or adaptive equipment, or both, can be the key to the child's independence.

IV.   What positioning and adaptive equipment do

A.   They allow for more normal movement by and for the child.

    1.   Muscle tone: amount of tension in a muscle or group of muscles.

        a.   Hypertonicity (high muscle tone)

            (1)   spasticity, rigidity
            (2)   feels like stiffness, making it difficult to move the joints
            (3)   sometimes is misinterpreted as being very strong

        b.   Hypotonicity (low muscle tone)

            (1)   feels like weakness or floppiness
            (2)   not enough muscle control to hold or support the body

        c.   Combination: the neck and trunk usually are hypotonic and the extremities are hypertonic

    2.   Reflexes: postures and movements the child cannot control

B.   Positioning and adaptive equipment can help to strengthen weak muscles.

C.   Positioning and adaptive equipment help to prevent joint tightness and contractures.

V.   Basic principles of positioning and adaptive equipment

A.   Caregivers should strive for a balance of

    1.   Flexion (bending) and extension (straightening).

    2.   Abduction (moving out) and adduction (moving in).

    3.   Rotation of child's torso helps achieve this balance.

    4.   Examples:

        a.   If a child's legs are always straight, bend one or both of them.

b.   If he/she arches the back, help him/her to bend or twist it.

c.   If the arms are bent out by the shoulders, help straighten them forward to the front of the body.

B.   Stability/mobility

    1.   Head control is the basis of trunk control.

    2.   The child's trunk (torso) has to have enough control or support so the head or extremities can move freely.

    3.   For the child to move, muscle tone must be relaxed or improved.

C.   To gain symmetry, the head, eyes and hands have to work together in the middle of the body, as opposed to reaching and playing primarily with one hand.

D.   Support should be given where needed, but the goal is to decrease and take away support as soon as possible; the amount of support needed may vary with the position and the difficulty of the task.

E.   "Key points" for support and handling are

    1.   neck/trunk,

    2.   shoulders and shoulder girdle, and

    3.   hips and pelvis.

F.   Using these key points when positioning a child helps caregivers to change the muscle tone and improve the child's posture and movements.

G.   Positioning prepares a child for functioning so he/she can do as much as he/she is capable of doing.

H.   Excessive effort by the child, and moving the child too rapidly, will increase abnormal tone and movements.

VI.   How to position the child

A.   Each child has his/her own specific problems. By asking the parents or therapist, caregivers can easily learn the specific techniques that are best for each individual child.

B.   These children cannot shift their weight well, so their position has to be changed frequently.

C.   What to use

    1.   almost anything — pillows, towels, blankets, your body

    2.   firm but pliable materials

    3.   readily cleanable materials

    4.   adaptive equipment from medical supply companies

    5.   products from toy stores, catalogs for infants/children and general merchandise stores for infants/children

    6.   items reflecting appropriate chronological age and developmental skill level

D.   Where and when to use positioning and adaptive equipment

    1.   Spending time on the floor gives children the opportunity to learn and practice movements.

    2.   Side-lying

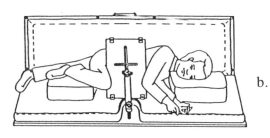

Figure 1
Side-lying position

        a.   Decreases neck and trunk extensor hypertonicity (arching), increases symmetry, brings hands together at mid-line, and increases eye/hand coordination.

        b.   Child is positioned on side with arms forward to mid-line, neck and trunk slightly flexed, and bottom leg straight, and top leg flexed.

        c.   Adaptive materials include manufactured or homemade foam or triwall sidelyers (Figure 1), pillows, beanbags, SIDS pillow.

3. On stomach (Figure 2)

 a. Positioning decreases hypertonicity in neck, trunk, and arms to make it easier for the child to raise the head and take weight on the arms or to play; also used to help decrease full body extension and to develop normal extension strength in the neck, trunk, and arms.

 b. The child is positioned on a raised surface so the head is unsupported, the chest is raised and supported, and the arms are slightly in front of shoulders, with forearms or hands on floor.

 c. Adaptations and material include rolled towel or blanket, pillow, wedge, Boppy™, or half-roll; prone boards (padded boards with wheels and safety straps) may be used for movement in this position.

Figure 2
Positioning child on a roll

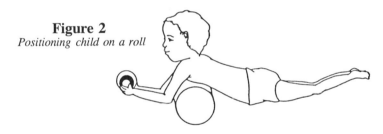

4. Back-lying

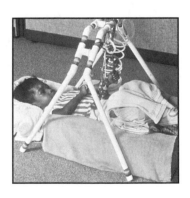

 a. Used to decrease hypertonicity or to improve posture and function of hypotonic infants and to develop strength in neck, leg, and trunk flexors.

 b. In this position the neck and trunk are flexed and arms forward, legs flexed and rolled out for high tone, or legs straight and close together for low tone.

 c. May use pillow, rolled towel, Boppy, or wedge, half-roll.

Back-lying

5. Sitting

    a. Basic principles for sitting in chairs

        (1) A chair should enable the child to achieve good head and trunk control so his/her arms may come forward for use of the hands.

        (2) The child's lower spine should be against the back of the chair, the hips bent at least to 90°, with knees also bent to 90°, and the feet flat on the floor or footrest when sitting upright.

        (3) Child should sit in the chair for only short periods.

        (4) Types of chairs

            (a) triwall
            (b) Tumbleform™
            (c) Kaye™ or Rifton™ adjustable chair
            (d) Educube™
            (e) box chair
            (f) Sassy Seat™ or table
            (g) Movable chairs, umbrella strollers, travel chairs, wheelchairs, caster carts

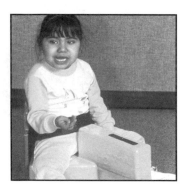

Tumbleform with child

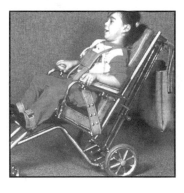

Travel chair

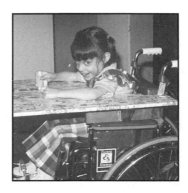

Wheelchair with tray

b. Adaptations for sitting in chairs (Figure 3)

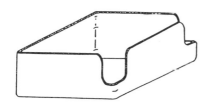

Figure 3

Adaptive chair made from a cardboard box

(1) side supports for head
(2) side supports for trunk
(3) abduction wedge to keep legs apart
(4) elevating the arms on a table or box about nipple height to help the child to sit up straight (Figure 4)
(5) tray attached to chair for play/support
(6) triwall (with or without tray) or wooden inserts in chairs
(7) rubber sink protector or dicem placed on chair seat to prevent slipping
(8) heads up (Figure 5)

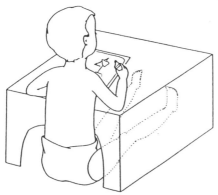

Figure 4

Cardboard box with table

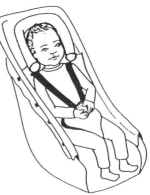

Figure 5

A "heads up"

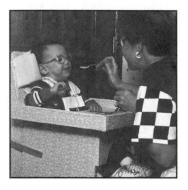

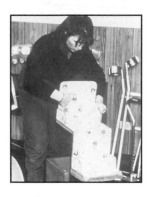

High-back triwall with tray   *Triwall insert in chair*

6.   Semi-reclining sitting

a.   The child should be positioned so the head is mid-line, shoulders and arms are forward, hips and knees are flexed, and the child is secured with safety straps.

b.   Types of chairs

(1)   bouncer (Figure 6)
(2)   infant seat
(3)   beanbag chair (Figure 7)
(4)   sofa corner
(5)   Tumbleform™ feeder seat reclined on wedge base
(6)   hammock

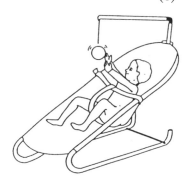

Figure 6
Bouncer

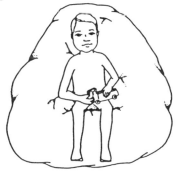

Figure 7
Beanbag chair

7.   Floor sitting

a.   The child's head and trunk should be supported where needed, with the arms forward.

b.   Undesirable floor-sitting positions

(1) *Sacral sitting:* weight is shifted back onto sacrum with upper back rounded rather than trunk erect with weight on bottom (Figure 8).

(2) *W-sitting:* sitting between legs and hips and knees bent and feet pointing behind (see Figure 9).

(3) *Tailor* (sometimes called Indian sitting or crossed-leg sitting) (Figure 10).

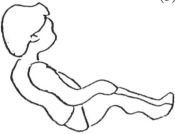

Figure 8
Sacral sitting

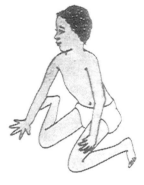

Figure 9
W-sitting

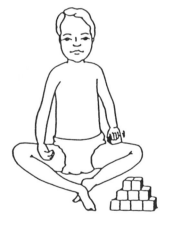

Figure 10
Tailor sitting

c.   Desirable floor-sitting position: side-sitting (Figure 11)

d.   The pelvis should be pulled back so the child sits on his/her bottom instead of rounded on his/her sacrum (tailbone), using the following supports:

(1) against sofa

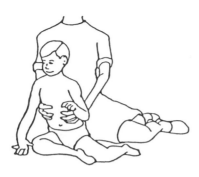

Figure 11
Side-sitting

(2)   supported by your legs
(3)   playpen
(4)   corner chair (Figure 12)
(5)   floor sitter (triwall)
(6)   Boppy™
(7)   Sassy Seat™
(8)   wall corner
(9)   box chair
(10)   box table

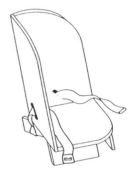

Figure 12
Corner chair

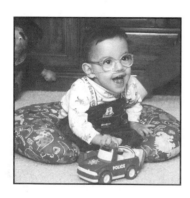

Child in Boppy™

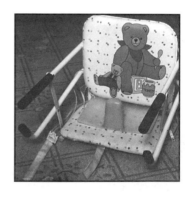

Sassy Seat™

8.   Kneeling[1]

    a.   Kneeling support has to be prevented from tipping
    b.   Use

        (1)   Educube
        (2)   bench
        (3)   fireplace hearth
        (4)   box

---

[1] Check with parent/guardian before having child kneel.

9. Standing[2]

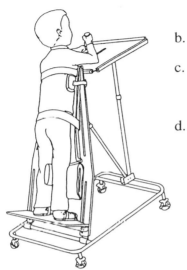

a. Putting children in a standing posture may be detrimental to the development of some children. This includes letting them stand on your lap when holding them over your shoulder.
b. Standing must be done in specific ways.
c. Use of walkers and Johnny Jump-Ups™ also can be harmful for children with motor (movement) problems.
d. Use

(1) couch/chair
(2) box
(3) bench
(4) barrel
(5) prone stander (may have wheels) (Figure 13)
(6) floor stander
(7) standing play table
(8) parapodium

Figure 13
Wheeled prone stander

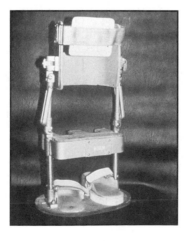

Parapodium

---

[2] Consult parent/guardian before standing a child.

10.   Walking: assistive devices

a.   Walkers

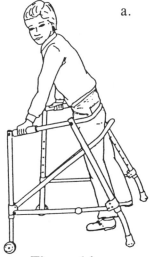

(1)   Rollator™: walker with wheels on the
       front two legs
(2)   Posterior walker: walker with metal
       frame behind the child and wheels on the
       front two legs (Figure 14).
(3)   Weighted toy shopping cart

Figure 14
Posterior walker

b.   Para-Aide™ (Figure 15)

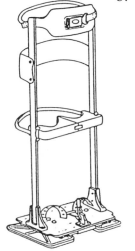

(1)   Supports child's trunk and legs in
       standing position
(2)   Usually for children with spina bifida or
       spinal cord injury
(3)   Allows child to stand and shift weight to
       walk

Figure 15
Swivel walker - Para-Aide

c. Crutches

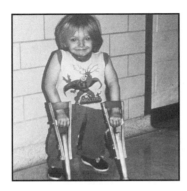

(1) Forearm crutches that have bands going around the forearms

(2) Axillary

(a) Traditional crutch that goes from under the armpit to the floor.
(b) weight borne on hands and not under the arms

Child using forearm crutches

VII. Orthoses (braces)

A. Custom-made for each individual child.

B. Materials are

1. plastic,

2. plastic and metal, or

3. metal and leather.

C. Instructions to get from parents/therapist:

1. how to take them on and off

2. when to use (which activities are enhanced or hampered by their use)

D. Post illustrations showing dos and don'ts, for quick reference.

E. May cause redness/sores (document and report to parent/guardian and therapist).

F. Types (named for the joints they cover; used to increase/decrease movement and promote stability).

1. Foot Orthosis (FO)

a. heel cup or foot support, or both
b. used to correct heel or foot position

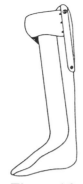

Ankle-Foot Orthosis (AFO) (Figure 16)

    a.   splint or brace from below the knee to the foot

    b.   may or may not have movable ankle joint

    c.   used to correct ankle/foot position and movement

Figure 16
Ankle-Foot Orthosis (AFO)

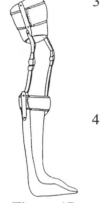

3.   Tone-Reducing Ankle-Foot Orthosis) (TRAFO)

    a.   splint designed to decrease lower extremity extensor tone to make standing and walking easier

    b.   corrects ankle/foot positioning and movement

4.   Knee-Ankle-Foot Orthosis (KAFO) (Figure 17)

    a.   splint or brace from above the knee down to the foot

    b.   knee joint may bend or lock straight

    c.   used to control knee/ankle/foot position and movement

Figure 17
Knee-Ankle-Foot Orthosis (KAFO)

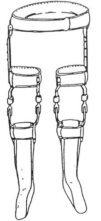

5.   Hip-Knee-Ankle-Foot Orthosis (HKAFO) (Figure 18)

    a.   splints or braces connected by a pelvic band that goes around the child's lower back

    b.   hip and knee joints may bend or lock

    c.   used to control position and movement of hips/knees/ankles/feet

Figure 18
Hip-Knee-Ankle-Foot Orthosis (HKAFO)

6. Reciprocating brace: HKAFO with cable attached that moves alternate legs as child shifts weight

7. Inhibitory casts (Figure 19)

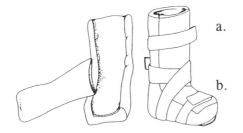

   a. plaster or synthetic casts used to decrease lower extremity extensor tone for better standing and walking

   b. usually come on and off by velcro straps

Figure 19
Inhibitory casts

8. Adaptive tennis shoes

   a. regular tennis shoes adapted by a therapist
   b. used to improve tone and foot positioning

9. Denis Browne splint

   a. two shoes connected and separated by a metal bar
   b. usually used to correct club feet

10. Pavlic harness

   a. a firm roll hooked between child's thighs with a cloth harness over the chest
   b. used to keep the legs apart to correct hip dislocations

VIII. Other assistive devices

A. Body jackets

   1. plastic-like jackets that fit securely around the child's trunk

   2. help correct scoliosis (curvature of the spine)

B. Prostheses (artificial limbs)

C. Helmets

   1. protect the head

2. used with children who have seizure problems, and sometimes with children who fall because of poor balance for children with seizure problems, or occasionally with those who fall because of poor balance

D. Hand splints

1. increase hand function

2. designed individually

3. commercial splints available

BIBLIOGRAPHY

Batshaw, M. L., & Perret, Y. M. (1992). *Children with handicaps: A medical primer* (ed.). Baltimore: Paul H. Brookes.

Bohannon, R., Mahoney, J., & Portnow, J. (1994). Self-help aids for minor disabilities. *Patient Care, 28*(5), 141-146, 151-154, 161-162.

Bowe, F. G. (1995). *Birth to five: Early childhood special education.* New York: Delmar.

Cook, A. M., & Hussey, S. M. (1995). *Assistive technologies: Principles and practice.* St. Louis: Mosby Year Book.

Laskowski, E. R. (1991). Snow skiing for the physically disabled. *Mayo Clinic Proceedings, 66*(2), 160-172.

Perr, A. (1993). Adaptive equipment: Freedom and independence for people with disabilities. *Journal of Religion in Disability and Rehabilitation, 1*(1), 81-87.

RESOURCES

American Physical Therapy Association (at First Start), 111 North Fairfax Street, Alexandria, VA 22314; (703) 684-2782

Independent Living Aids, 27 East Mall, Plainview, NY 11803; (516) 752-8080

National Parent Network on Disabilities (Toys tested by Toy Tips®

Physically Impaired Association of Michigan (PAM), Assistance Centre, 601 West Maple Street, Lansing, MI 48906-5038; 1-800-274-7426

CHILD ABUSE AND NEGLECT

I.   **Definitions**

   A.   Physical abuse: an act of bodily harm inflicted intentionally.

   B.   Sexual abuse: exposure to sexual experiences to which the child cannot consent or sexual experiences that are not developmentally appropriate.

   C.   Emotional neglect and psychological maltreatment: lack of attention and love; negative and hostile verbal and nonverbal treatment.

   D.   Physical neglect: failure of the caregiver to provide adequate food, clothing shelter, medical care, or supervision.

II. **Prevalence of child abuse and neglect**[1]

   A.   Approximately 3 million reports of child abuse and neglect were recorded in 1993, of which more than a million were confirmed.

   B.   The breakdown of all types of confirmed cases of abuse is as follows:

Physical Abuse	22.3%
Sexual abuse	13.6%
Neglect	49.9%
Emotional abuse	5.1%
Other abuse	9.1%

   C.   In 46% of the cases, the children were under age 3, and 86% of the cases involved children under age 5.

   D.   In 1993, about three children in the United States died daily as a result of child abuse or neglect.

III. **Responsibility to report.**   Virtually every state has child protection laws that identify professionals and others who are mandated to report suspected child abuse or neglect.   Child care workers and preschool teachers usually are included in those laws.   Failure to report abuse or neglect usually entails

---

[1] From *The State of America's Children Yearbook: 1995*, by the Children's Defense Fund, Washington, DC, 1995. The statistics are based on 1993 data.

misdemeanor criminal charges for mandated reporters, and may make the professional who failed to report pay the costs of subsequent injuries to the child.

A.   Each state has a "children's code" that defines what constitutes child abuse and neglect for purposes of juvenile or family court protection proceedings. A copy of this law may be obtained from your state or local social service agency. Most states also identify who is regarded as a mandated reporter.

B.   In addition to reports by mandated reporters, most states will investigate reports of suspected abuse or neglect from other concerned callers.

C.   Caregivers should inquire about the child care center's policy for reporting abuse/neglect. Every child care center should have a policy that is shared with parents/guardians as they enroll their children.

D.   Caregivers should discuss with a professional in the investigating agency when and what to say to parents/guardians.

E.   Common sense should be used in the decision to report. If a child is injured on a single occasion, the child and the parent/guardian should be asked how it occurred. There may be a reasonable explanation. Repeated "reasonable" instances or explanations that don't fit the injury are grounds for suspicion.

F.   When making a report to the criminal or child protection system, description of physical indicators of abuse (what you see), behavioral indicators (how the child acts), and your observations of parents/guardians are helpful.

G.   All relevant information should be documented in writing. Keep a copy for yourself.

IV.   **Risk factors.** Early intervention is the most effective way to stop a destructive pattern of parenting. Risk factors *may* include the following:

A.   Characteristics of the parent/guardian

    1.   Parent's/guardian's own history of abuse, neglect, or maltreatment

    2.   Young age of parent/guardian

      3.   Parent's/guardian's history of alcohol or drug abuse

      4.   Parent's/guardian's low self-esteem

  B.   Characteristics of the child and the relationship with parent/guardian

      1.   A child with special needs or one who poses special challenges

      2.   Overly high expectations for the child by the parent/guardian

      3.   A parent/guardian regarding the child as "different"

      4.   The parent/guardian being apathetic or nonresponsive to child

  C.   Circumstances

      1.   No visible support system

      2.   Parent/guardian under a lot of stress

V.   **Indications of child abuse and neglect.**[2] Abuse and neglect cannot be identified by race, ethnicity or socioeconomic class. Children are potential victims because of their vulnerable, powerless position. Many of the indicators, behaviors, and risk factors listed below may be natural, normal responses for any child. When several of these behaviors are consistent over time and pervasive, however, they are cause for concern.[3]

  A.   Physical neglect

      1.   Physical indicators (child)

          a.   consistent hunger/malnutrition, poor hygiene
          b.   excessive responsibility for younger siblings
          c.   clothes dirty or wrong for the weather
          d.   comes to school without breakfast

---

[2] Indicators of abuse and neglect were provided by C. Henry Kempe National Center for the Prevention and Treatment of Child Abuse and Neglect, Denver, CO.

[3] Source: *Personal Health: A Multicultural Approach,* by Patricia A. Floyd, Sandra E. Mimms, and Caroline Yelding-Howard (Englewood, CO: Morton Publishing, 1995), p. 81.

      e.   consistent lack of supervision, especially in dangerous activities or for long periods; latchkey children

      f.   often tired, no energy

      g.   unattended physical problems or medical needs

      h.   infants with a noticeably flat head, or bald spot

      i.   abandonment

      j.   emaciated, distended stomach

      k.   nonorganic failure to thrive

2.   Behavioral indicators (child)

      a.   low self-esteem

      b.   a variety of developmental delays (cognitive, language, motor, social, emotional, self-help)

      c.   behavior extremes

      d.   destructive to self and/or others

      e.   difficulty following rules; vandalism

      f.   self-stimulating behaviors

      g.   begs, steals food

      h.   craves affection

      i.   frequently absent or tardy

      j.   extended stays at school (early arrival and late departure)

      k.   constant fatigue, listlessness, falls asleep in class

      l.   depressed/apathetic

      m.   signs of alcohol or drug use

      n.   states there is no caretaker at home

      o.   sexual misconduct

      p.   repeated ingestion of harmful substances

      q.   excessive child care and housework responsibilities

      r.   role reversal ("mothers" the parent/guardian)

      s.   unable to play

      t.   disassociation; "always daydreaming"

3.   Observations of parent/guardian

      a.   low self-esteem

      b.   misuses drugs/alcohol

      c.   history of neglect as a child

      d.   parent's/guardian's needs come before child's

      e.   isolated from friends, relatives, neighbors; lacks social skills

      f.   chaotic home life (disorganized, upset)

      g.   needy

      h.   overwhelmed and depressed

      i.   tired, dirty, unkempt

       j.   unsafe living conditions (no food in home; garbage and excrement in living areas, exposed wiring, drugs and poisons within reach of children)

       k.   flat affect (emotionless): lacks motivation, lethargic, passive, indifferent

       l.   teen parent, parent with mental illness, parent with mental retardation

B.   Physical abuse

    1.   Physical indicators (child)

       a.   frequent injuries, usually explained as accidental

       b.   unexplained, suspicious, or recurrent bruises and welts

           (1)   on face, lips, mouth
           (2)   on torso, back, buttocks, thighs
           (3)   in various stages of healing
           (4)   clustered, forming regular or unusual patterns (nail scratches, bite marks)
           (5)   reflecting shape of article used to inflict (electric cord, belt buckle, hand)
           (6)   on several different surface areas
           (7)   appear regularly after absence, weekend, or vacation

       c.   unexplained, suspicious burns

           (1)   cigarette or cigar burns, especially on soles, palms, back, buttocks
           (2)   immersion burns (sock-like, glove-like, doughnut-shaped on buttocks or genitalia)
           (3)   patterns like electric burner, iron, etc.
           (4)   rope burns on arms, legs, neck, or torso

       d.   unexplained or suspicious fractures, sprains, dislocations

           (1)   restricted range of motion
           (2)   to skull, nose, facial structure
           (3)   in various stages of healing
           (4)   multiple or spiral fractures
           (5)   bucket handle fractures (to the growth plate)
           (6)   chip fractures

e.   unexplained or suspicious lacerations or abrasions

    (1)   to mouth, lips, gums, eyes
    (2)   to external genitalia

f.   missing teeth
g.   human bite marks
h.   bald spots

2.   Behavioral indicators (child)

a.   low self-esteem
b.   poor eye contact
c.   behavioral extremes

    (1)   aggressiveness (hits, kicks, bites; is defiant, demanding; causes trouble or interferes with others; breaks or damages property; is destructive to self or others, or both)
    (2)   withdrawal (usually shy, avoids other people including children, seems too anxious to please, seems too ready to let other people say and do things to him/her without protest)

d.   may evidence a variety of developmental delays (cognitive, language, motor, social, emotional, self-help)
e.   child's story of how a physical injury occurred is not believable; doesn't seem to fit the type or seriousness of the injury observed; reports injury by parent/guardian
f.   flinches from touch
g.   hypervigilant (always on guard)
h.   apprehensive when other children cry
i.   cries easily and often, showing no real expectation of being comforted
j.   seems frightened of parent/guardian or shows little or no distress at being separated from parent/guardian
k.   is afraid to go home or avoids home (consistently arrives at school early or leaves late)
l.   assumes parental role and may be very protective toward abusive parent
m.   continually seeks attention, favors, food, or affection from any adult

n.   accident-prone, moves awkwardly
o.   complains of soreness
p.   wears clothing inappropriate for the weather to cover body
q.   child's attention wanders, and easily becomes self-absorbed

3.   Observations of parent/guardian

a.   has history of abuse as a child
b.   misuses drugs/alcohol
c.   has low self-esteem
d.   depressed, lonely, isolated, no support system
e.   parent's/guardian's needs come before child's; unaware of how to fulfill their own emotional needs and expect child to fill adult's emotional void
f.   inappropriate developmental expectations of child's behaviors; may expect adult behavior
g.   domestic violence
h.   rigid, compulsive; continuous, underlying anger
i.   child reminds parents/guardians of someone they hate (often themselves) or parent/guardian sees child as "bad," "evil," a "monster," "witch," "difficult," "different," "hard to manage"
j.   shows signs of lack of control or fear of losing control
k.   seems unconcerned about the child
l.   offers illogical, unconvincing, contradictory explanations or has no explanation for the child's injury
m.   attempts to conceal the child's injury or to protect the identity of the person(s) responsible
n.   lacks warmth in interactions with child
o.   extremely critical and demanding of child
p.   believes in harsh physical punishment as the only real way to discipline with an undue fear of "spoiling" the child; discipline not consistent with child's age, condition, or behavior
q.   ignores the child's crying or reacts with extreme impatience
r.   harshly pulls or pushes the child

C.   Sexual abuse[4]

    1.   Physical indicators (often no visible indicators)

        a.   torn, stained, or bloody underclothing
        b.   pain, itching, red, or swollen in genital area
        c.   odor in genital area
        d.   semen around the genitals or on clothing
        e.   lacerations, bruises, or bleeding in external genitalia or anal area
        f.   poor sphincter control
        g.   frequent urinary or yeast infections
        h.   eating problems: sudden weight gain, loss of appetite, gagging, vomiting
        i.   frequent, unexplained sore throat
        j.   sexually transmitted disease
        k.   newly acquired bodily complaints (stomach aches, headaches, genital pain, encopresis [involuntary passing of feces], enuresis [bedwetting], unexplained fatigue)
        l.   infections of the mouth, gums, or throat. (Be vigilant for sexually transmitted diseases of anus or throat.)
        m.   difficulty with walking or sitting

    2.   Behavioral indicators (child)

        a.   poor self-esteem
        b.   may show developmental delays
        c.   self-destructive; may engage in self-mutilation such as sticking self with pins or cutting self with sharp objects
        d.   abrupt change in child's behavior: moodiness, aggressiveness, withdrawal, depression, excessive crying or daydreaming, feelings of shame or guilt, irritability, crankiness, short-tempered behavior, appears withdrawn or engages in fantasy or baby-like behavior; regressive behaviors (wetting pants, thumbsucking, rocking), smearing feces (subsequent to toilet training)
        e.   poor hygiene or compulsive cleanliness
        f.   abruptly avoids activity that was formerly enjoyed

---

[4]   Please note that no one indicator would confirm child sexual abuse but identification of several should cause suspicion.

g. bizarre, sophisticated, or unusual sexual behavior or knowledge (oral, vaginal, anal penetration of dolls, animals, children; attempts to expose others' genitals, manifestations of unusual sexual behaviors or themes through child's drawings, stories, poems, schoolwork)

h. persistent, inappropriate, seductive, promiscuous behavior toward peers or adults including excessive or compulsive masturbation

i. extreme modesty or fear of sexual issues, secretive behavior

j. change in affect (emotional behavior) or body language when a certain adult is discussed; afraid to be alone with adults, especially males; makes indirect allusions to or reports sexual assault

k. frequent absences from school, many times justified by parent/guardian

l. mistrustful, threatened by physical contact or closeness

m. role reversal, overly concerned for siblings

n. sudden fears, phobias, and anxieties; overt anger; compulsivity; hysteria and lack of emotional control; needs more reassurance than usual; clings to parent/guardian

o. sleep disturbances (nightmares, fear of going to bed, wanting light on, waking up during night, fear of sleeping alone)

p. firesetting, tortures animals

3. Observations of parent

a. history of sexual abuse as a child
b. low self-esteem
c. misuses drugs/alcohol
d. geographically isolated; isolation/alienation of child and family members within the community
e. role reversal and blurred boundaries
f. over-involved father and passive-dependent mother
g. extremely controlling, overprotective and jealous of child
h. appears to be "okay" to others (friends, co-workers)
i. inadequate coping skills
j. loss of spouse through death or divorce
k. frequent absences from home by one of the parents/guardians

        l.   mother absent, disabled, ill, or unavailable
        m.   rigid, restrictive home environment
        n.   presence of a stepfather
        o.   parental conflict

D.   Psychological maltreatment (often occurs in conjunction with physical or sexual abuse or neglect)

    1.   Physical indicators (often no visible indicators)

        a.   physical manifestations of nervous disorders (overweight, underweight, skin rashes, headaches, stomach aches, asthma, severe allergies)
        b.   nonorganic failure to thrive in association with feeding disorders
        c.   hopeless, empty look

    2.   Behavioral indicators (child)

        a.   low self-esteem
        b.   behavior extremes

            (1)   compliant, passive
            (2)   aggressive, demanding, disruptive

        c.   overly adaptive behavior

            (1)   inappropriately adult-like
            (2)   inappropriately infantile

        d.   may evidence developmental delays (cognitive, language, motor, social, emotional, self-help)
        e.   speech disorders such as stuttering
        f.   self-destructive/suicidal
        g.   increased anxiety
        h.   habit disorders (sucking, biting, rocking)
        i.   regressive behaviors (bedwetting, thumbsucking)
        j.   withdrawn, apathetic, depressed
        k.   antisocial, destructive
        l.   substance abuse
        m.   eating disorders
        n.   sleep disorders such as insomnia
        o.   craves affection

3. Observations of parent

    a.   history of maltreatment
    b.   low self-esteem
    c.   misuses drugs/alcohol
    d.   unrealistic expectations
    e.   frequent blaming or belittling of child
    f.   perceives child as bad, evil
    g.   treats children in family unequally
    h.   cold and rejecting
    i.   withholds love
    j.   lacks nurturing skills
    k.   passive/aggressive behaviors
    l.   ignores child
    m.   isolates child from social interactions
    n.   mental illness

VI. Special care needs

A. Provide for the child's emotional and developmental needs.

B. Help the children feel comfortable with their bodies.

C. Provide for the safety and security of all children in your care, as even young children can harm their peers physically or sexually.

D. Establish a "no secrets" rule. Secrets protect perpetrators. Teach children the difference between a *secret* and a surprise, and behaviors that are *private*.

E. Continue to communicate with parent/guardian and social worker regarding the child's progress.

F. Look for strengths in the parent/guardian, and strive to develop a positive relationship.

G. Develop a list of resources that might be helpful to the parent/guardian.

BIBLIOGRAPHY

Behrman, R. E. (Ed.) (1994). Sexual abuse of children, *The future of children,* 4(2). (A periodical of the Center for the Future of Children, the David and Lucille Packard Foundation.)

Besharov, D. (1995). *The state of America's children yearbook: 1995.* Washington, DC: Children's Defense Fund.

Besharov, D. (1990). *Recognizing child abuse.* New York: Free Press.

RESOURCES

Hotlines

American Humane Association, Children's Division (Denver): 1-800-227-4645

Clearinghouse for Child Abuse and Neglect (Washington, DC): 1-800-394-3366

Family Violence Prevention Fund: 1-800-777-1960

National Committee to Prevent Child Abuse (Chicago): (312) 663-3520

National Victim Center: 1-800-FYI-CALL

Videos and Booklets (available from Kempe National Center, 1205 Oneida Street, Denver, CO 80220; (303) 321-3963):

- The Theft of Childhood
- Nobody's Home (on neglect)
- Identifying, Reporting and Handling Disclosure of the Sexually Abused Child
- Child Abuse: Breaking the Cycle

OBSERVATION AND RECORDING

I. Record keeping requirements

A. The type of records a child care facility may be required to keep varies by state and the size and nature of the center.

   1. Requirements vary by states and locality.

   2. Any time caregivers administer medicine, the time, the amount, and the person giving the medicine should be recorded.[1]

B. The administrator of a child care facility should contact state and local regulatory bodies to determine the applicable requirements and guidelines.

C. In many centers, the forms for observing and recording a child's behavior are kept on file at the center, along with reports to parents.

D. Types of information to be included in a suitable record-keeping system are available from sources including those listed in the Resources.

II. Importance of accurate and objective recording

A. Careful observation and recording can improve the quality of child care.

B. Observation and recording can document a child's physical, cognitive, and emotional development.

C. Observation and recording assist in

   1. discovering of a child's capabilities,

   2. program planning,

---

[1] Administration of medication is generally regarded as an invasive procedure and, as such, is a nursing task that may be subject to statutory provisions or to regulations established by your State's Nursing Board. If this is the case, legislation or regulatory guidelines may be in place that determine whether or not and how this task may be delegated to a non-health-licensed individual (other than the child's parent or guardian). For the safety of the children, and due to the risk of personal and agency liability, you are urged to contact your State Board of Nursing to inquire about the status of delegation of invasive procedures in your state.

3. communicating better with parents/guardians,

4. identifying children with special needs, and

5. accountability.

D. Observations in child-care settings provide a real-life sample of a child's development.

III. Participation by Caregivers

A. A caregiver may be called upon to observe and record, for example, when

1. a child has difficulty adjusting to child care,

2. a child has a problem behavior,

3. parents/guardians want information on a child's progress,

4. a child seems to be developing slowly, or

5. complying with a child's therapy program.

B. Objective, complete records are needed to make accurate reports.

IV. Observation

A. Observation may help identify learning experiences, keyed to the child's developmental level.

B. Observation provides specific information on individual child.

C. Observation may be made in interactions with a single child or during small-group activities.

D. Considerations when observing a child:

1. Why is the observation being done?

2. Who or what is being observed?

3. Which behaviors are of interest? When? Where?

4. What information do you need to answer the previous questions? How will the information be used? How should it be recorded and how often?

5. What does observation ultimately do for the child?

E. Accurate and objective observations require that the caregiver:

1. Understand normal child growth and development.

2. Observe the child's developmental level in comparison to his/her peers.

   a. What is the observed child doing? What are other children of the same age doing?
   b. How does the child interact with familiar children and adults?
   c. Should the observation be made at another time? With other children and adults present? With other toys and materials available? While other activities are going on?

F. When observing a child's behavior, notice

1. the child's motor actions (running, for example),

2. the child's verbal actions (such as screaming or whispering),

3. the child's ease and rate of performing an activity,

4. whether the child completes or abandons the activity, and

5. how long the child persists in the activity.

V. Recording

A. Efficient record-keeping provides documentation of events and promotes accurate communication among caregivers, parents, and providers of services to children.

B.   In many settings a card system is the preferred recording method. The cards for each child are stored in a file. Other methods are available, too, such as anecdotal descriptions, logs, time samples, checklists and rating scales, tape or video recordings (parent permission may be required), portfolios (representative samples of a child's work), communication notebooks, and summary reports.

C.   Caregivers should record actual happenings, not emotional reactions to them, and avoid labeling the behavior and expressing judgments and opinions. As examples:

1.   Write, "Johnny ran to the book corner, buried his head in a pillow, and cried loudly," rather than, "Johnny seemed very upset and sad."

2.   Write, "Mary ate 2 spoonsful of applesauce and drank 4 ounces of milk from a bottle" rather than, "Mary didn't seem very hungry today. She hardly ate anything."

VI.   **Implications for children with special needs**

A.   Examining and testing children with special needs again and again often focuses on the child's limits and can be unpleasant for the child.

B.   Observation can focus on a child's strengths and abilities and can be done while the child is involved in more pleasant activities.

C.   Play is an excellent, often overlooked means for observing children with special needs, during which a wide range abilities can be studied.

D.   Describing skills demonstrated in day-to-day child care activities may provide a well rounded picture of the child with special needs.

VII.   **Responsibilities of parents/guardians and caregivers**

A.   The parents/guardian should provide caregivers with the following information and instructions and update it as the child's needs change. In all cases below, the instructions should clearly identify the name of the child and the date the instructions were recorded.

1.   Feeding instructions

a. allergies (if any)
b. formula (brand, bottle or cup, warm or cold)
c. food: type (baby, junior, or table); self-feeding (fingers or spoon)
d. number of feedings when at center
e. any special instructions

2. Sleep instructions

a. special instructions such as use of pacifier, toy, or blanket
b. preferred sleep position

3. Medication request[2]

a. name of person making the request
b. medicine
c. dosage
d. reason for taking medicine
e. amount of medicine left in bottle
f. storage place
g. method of administration
h. time(s) to be given
i. suggestions for giving
j. side effects
k. signatures (parents and prescribing health professional)
l. duration (such as 1 week, 10 days, until finished)

4. Diapering instructions

a. brand of diapers
b. allergies (description)
c. type(s) of lotion, ointment, powder to use, if any, and circumstances of use (such as when the child is wet, has a bowel movement, has a rash)
d. special instructions

5. Special care request

a. reason for the request
b. request
c. instructions

---

[2] See footnote 1.

        d.   demonstration of procedure (what was demonstrated, by whom, and to whom)

        e.   requesting health professional (name and profession)

        f.   signed permission by parent/guardian to release information related to request (identifying child, request, and recipient of information)

B.   Sign out

    1.   Children should not leave the child-care center with anyone except the parent/guardian without documented permission by the parent/guardian.

    2.   The form should be signed by the parent/guardian and should identify the child, date of the request, and name(s) of person(s) permitted to sign the child out of the center.

C.   Caregivers are responsible for recording specific information on a daily report for the parent/guardian.

    1.   The daily report is an efficient means of logging observations and complying with parental instructions.

    2.   A copy should be kept on file.

    3.   The daily report should identify the child and the date of the report and should log actions and observations such as

        a.   feedings (times, types of food, amounts).

        b.   naps (times, length, comment).

        c.   medications administered[3] (times, medicine, dosage, person administering medication).

        d.   child's disposition (such as active, happy, cranky).

        e.   child's activities during the day.

        f.   outside care (such as going to a doctor's appointment or therapy session).

        g.   other comments about the child or events of the day.

---

[3]   See footnote 1.

4. Importance of daily report

    a. Parent/guardian knows what happened during the day.

    b. Parent/guardian can take appropriate action at home in regard to naps, food, medication, and the like.

    c. The report helps build trust between parent/ guardian and caregiver.

    d. The report provides an accurate record if needed in the future.

5. The report can be completed while children are napping or at a regularly scheduled time when another caregiver or aide covers responsibilities.

D. Other recording and reporting tools that may be helpful

1. Masterboard (a large chalkboard, dry-erase board, or similar large writing surface)

    a. may include any important information and may be helpful in filling out daily reports and organizing the center activities.

    b. can be used for an entire center or for a section (infant, toddler, or preschool section).

    c. provides information for all caregivers and can be useful when writing the daily report.

    d. may be tailored to the needs and activities of the group of children served but at a minimum should include the time of the event and all information necessary to document compliance with parental instructions.

2. Diapering board (sheet of paper posted in diapering area)

    a. useful in filling in the daily report and keeping track of any problems (for example, diarrhea) of which the staff and parent need to be aware.

    b. lists the names of children diapered during the day and such observations as:

        (1) time of each child's diaper change.

        (2) condition of the diaper (wet or bowel movement).

        (3) any problems (such as diarrhea, rashes).

3. Special care board to log the performance of any special requests; should identify each child receiving a special procedure, along with

   a. time of special procedure.
   b. type of activity.
   c. checkout and return times if the special procedure was provided by a professional outside of the room.
   d. descriptions of how the child participated with other children (if in an inclusive service).
   e. special instructions followed.

BIBLIOGRAPHY

Bergan, J. R., & Feld, J. K. (1993). Developmental assessment: New directions. *Young Children, 48*(5), 41-47.

Giek, K. A. (1992). Monitoring student progress through efficient record keeping. *Teaching Exceptional Children, 24*(3), 22-26.

Hills, T. W. (1993). Assessment in context: Teachers and children at work. *Young Children, 48*(5), 20-28.

Weber, C., Behl, D., & Summers, M. (1994). Watch them play — watch them learn. *Teaching Exceptional Children, 27*(1), 30-35.

RESOURCES

National Health and Safety Performance Standards: Guidelines for Out-of-Home Child Care, prepared by the American Public Health Association and American Academy of Pediatrics, edited and reproduced by the National Center for Education in Maternal and Child Health (NCEMCH) at Georgetown University in cooperation with the Maternal and Child Health Bureau.

For more information contact National Center for Education in Maternal and Child Health, 2000-15th Street North, Suite 701, Arlington, VA 22201-2617; (703) 524-7802

IV. COMMUNICATION AND COMMUNITY SUPPORT

Attitudes Toward Children with Disabilities and Chronic Conditions

Family Dynamics

Inclusion

Implications of Poverty

Legal Issues

Respecting Diversity

ATTITUDES TOWARD CHILDREN WITH DISABILITIES AND CHRONIC CONDITIONS

I. **Definition of disability**

   A. A person with a disability is defined here as one who has an impairment that affects his/her ability to see, hear, walk, talk, breathe, learn or work.

   B. Previous legislative definition used the term "handicap," which describes the consequences of a disability. If a disability doesn't hamper a person in daily life, it is not a handicap.

II. **Qualities of attitudes**

   A. Attitudes are acquired, not inborn.

      1. Attitudes represent values and beliefs.

      2. Attitudes consist of knowledge, feelings, and actions toward an individual, group, or subject.

   B Attitudes are based in part upon the amount and quality of information.

   C. Attitudes may be influenced by gaining more or different information.

   D. Attitudes are conveyed through words and phrases.

      1. Negative words and phrases

         a. Language that focuses on the disability may make the disability more important than the person as a human being.
         b. Negative words and phrases create a set of expectations that limit the child's opportunities and achievements.
         c. Negative words and phrases fail to reflect the individuality, equality, and dignity of children with special needs.

      2. Positive words and phrases

         a. Positive language helps to portray children with disabilities and chronic conditions more accurately.

b.   Positive words and phrases can help change negative attitudes about children with disabilities by focusing on the child as a person rather than on the disability or conditions.

c.   Positive words and phrases indicate that children with special needs are like other children in that children with and without disabilities have a full range of personality traits and characteristics.

III.   Sources and expression of negative attitudes

A.   Negative attitudes often arise when a person has:

1.   Limited knowledge about disabilities.

2.   Little or no experience in the company of people with disabilities.

B.   People without disabilities might reject children with special needs because:

1.   These children differ from the "ideal" child or what this society values.

2.   People may fear the disability (for example, HIV).

3.   People feel uncomfortable or intensely aware of what is different about the child and may think they don't know how to act toward the child.

C.   TV, newspapers, and movies can contribute to negative attitudes. People with special needs rarely are portrayed as ordinary or successful in socially valued ways.

D.   Some people have negative attitudes because they need to feel superior to other people.

E.   Children with disabilities often are seen as less capable, stable, or likeable than children without disabilities.

F.   Negative attitudes towards people with disabilities may be expressed through

1.   *Stereotyping:*   assuming that all people with disabilities are alike.

2.   *Patronizing:*   "talking down" to a person.

3.   *Overpraising:* overreacting to minor achievements (usually because expectations for the person are very low).

4.   *Labeling:* putting the disability before the person (for example, "Down syndrome child" versus "child with Down syndrome").

5.   *Rejecting close relationships* with children who have disabilities.

IV.   **Creating positive attitudes toward children with special needs**

A.   Correct information may:

1.   Reduce fears about people with the conditions.

2.   Remove barriers to knowing the person who has the condition.

3.   Make a person aware of the similarities between children with and without disabilities.

4.   Help a person examine his or her ideas or beliefs toward people with chronic conditions/disabilities.

B.   Experience with children with disabilities may help caregivers feel more comfortable in interacting with these children. Through experience a person may learn that children with disabilities:

1.   Are more similar to than different from other children.

2.   Are individuals.

C.   Legislative efforts alone will not alter attitudes.

1.   Positive attitudinal changes require changes in values and beliefs.

2.   Attitudes do not always change for the better, and positive changes do not always last.

D.   Inclusive child care settings usually offer advantages to all children.

1.   Children with disabilities can interact with children without disabilities.

2.   Children without disabilities learn to appreciate diversity and have a better understanding of whatever disabilities are present. This may promote acceptance of children with disabilities.

V.   Special care needs

A.   Treat infants, toddlers, and young children as *children*, whether they do or do not have a disability.

B.   Become "disability-blind"; do not focus on the disability.

C.   Help all children, regardless of their special needs, acquire a positive self-concept.

D.   Work as a partner with children with special needs and their parents/guardians, instead of working for or against them.

E.   If a child does not make the progress you expected, do not blame or reject the child. Infants, toddlers, and young children with disabilities need consistent warmth and acceptance.

F.   Encourage children with disabilities to participate as much as possible with their peers who do not have disabilities.

G.   Show respect toward children with disabilities.

H.   Nurture all children's physical, emotional, social, and intellectual development.

I.   Use fair guidance and disciplinary measures with children with and without disabilities alike.

BIBLIOGRAPHY

Anderson, R. J., & Antonak, R. F. (1992). The influence of attitudes and contact on reactions to persons with physical and speech disabilities. *Rehabilitation Counseling Bulletin, 35*(4), 240-242.

Eichinger, J., Rizzo, T., & Sirotnik, B. (1991). Changing attitudes toward people with disabilities. *Teacher Education and Special Education, 14*(2), 121-126.

Havranek, J. E. (1991). The social and individual costs of negative attitudes toward persons with physical disabilities. *Journal of Applied Rehabilitation Counseling, 22*(1), 15-21.

Soder, M. (1990). Prejudice or ambivalence? Attitudes toward persons with disabilities. *Disability, Handicap & Society, 5*(3), 227-241.

RESOURCES

Research and Training Center for Independent Living, *Guidelines for Reporting and Writing About People with Disabilities,* University of Kansas, Lawrence, KS

Rocky Mountain Region Disability & Business Technical Assistance Center, 3630 Sinton Rd., Suite 103, Colorado Springs, CO 80907 (*ADA Today,* edited by J. Hume)

FAMILY DYNAMICS

I. **Nature of families**

    A. Definition of "family"

        1. Any group of individuals may define themselves as a family and take on family obligations and responsibilities for one another.

        2. Individuals become part of a family by marriage, birth, adoption, or mutual consent.

        3. Family members may or may not reside in the same household.

    B. Types of families

        1. Traditional family: biological parents and their child(ren).

        2. Single-adult parents living alone or with others who are not related to the child.

        3. Married or unmarried teenage parents rearing their children with the assistance of their own extended family.

        4. One or both parents rearing their children in shared living arrangements.

        5. Married couple rearing children from one or both previous marriages.

        6. Single or married individuals rearing foster children.

        7. Single or married individuals rearing adopted children.

        8. Grandparent(s) rearing child(ren) in the absence of the parent(s).

        9. Extended families living in one home.

    C. Commonalities among families

        1. Family interactions

            a. A family is dynamic--constantly changing.
            b. A family is an interactive unit.

          (1)   Actions affecting any one member affect all members.

          (2)   Change in one family member's behavior has some impact on the other family members.

    c.   All family behaviors serve the family in some way. When families are under stress, they try to solve problems using methods they have used before.

    d.   How well the family works as a unit contributes to each member's individual health, well-being, and competence.

2.   Family tasks

    a.   Meeting the basic needs of the family for food, health care, shelter, and money.

    b.   Helping each family member to develop his/her own capabilities.

    c.   Providing emotional support to all family members.

    d.   Maintaining and changing relationships within the family to meet changing needs.

    e.   Participating in the community.

3.   Developmental stages (the changing relationships within a family as the family moves through the life cycle). These tend to follow a sequence like this:

    a.   couple without children
    b.   childbearing
    c.   preschool
    d.   school-age
    e.   teenage
    f.   young adults becoming independent
    g.   parents in an empty nest
    h.   aging family members

D.   Differences between families

1.   Social and cultural characteristics

    a.   A family's beliefs and practices in childrearing are influenced by culture and environment.

b. Cultural, racial, ethnic, or religious background may strongly influence how a family reacts to and copes with illness. Families may differ in

(1) ways of behaving when health problems arise,
(2) the meanings they attribute to a child's illness or disability,
(3) interpretation or expression of symptoms, and
(4) how, when, or from whom they seek help.

2. Economic level

3. Parental behavior toward a child as influenced by

a. age
b. sex
c. marital/partnership status
d. experience with parenting
e. education
f. employment
g. individual personality

E. Roles and responsibility

1. Each family member, and the family as a whole, is expected to perform certain tasks.

a. The age and sex of each family member may determine his/her role and function.
b. Family members have differing abilities to fulfill or change their roles.

2. When a chronic health problem or disability is present, family members may have to change their roles.

II. Effects of diagnosis on families

A. Families have many different reactions to diagnosis of a child's disability or chronic condition. Most go through a period of adjustment.

1. There is no single pattern of emotional response.

2.   Reactions and feelings of family members often co-exist; individual family members may have different feelings at any given point.

3.   Changes in the diagnosis or new diagnoses may require families to readjust to the new information.

4.   As the child faces new developmental challenges or as the complications of a chronic condition unfold, the family may have new emotions or may re-experience previous emotional reactions.

B.   Emotional responses to diagnosis of a chronic condition or disability (in general chronological order)

1.   Shock: a time of disorganization, panic, distress; often not able to understand information.

2.   Denial: refusal to believe information about their child.

3.   Anger or projection of blame: may be directed toward medical personnel, mate, or other family members, God, or the child.

4.   Depression/sadness: loss of a "dream," feeling hopeless about the future.

5.   Guilt: concern of family members that somehow they have caused the problem.

6.   Rejection: directed at the child, the medical profession, or toward other family members.

7.   Withdrawal: a coping tool in which the person does not reveal his/her thoughts and feelings.

8.   Isolation: avoiding situations, shunning others, or complaining of being alone, lonely, rejected, or unwanted.

9.   Confusion: mixed thoughts, emotions; disturbed sleep.

10.   Worry: anxious; may seem preoccupied or lost in thought; asks a lot of questions.

11. Acceptance: emotionally embracing the child who has unique strengths and limitations; also, accepting the family's role in the child's life.

C. Differences in family members' reactions

    1. Parents' reactions

        a. Mothers and fathers may perceive family needs differently.
        b. Fathers and mothers may rely on different coping strategies.
        c. A father's acceptance is instrumental in family acceptance.

    2. Siblings may

        a. identify with the child,
        b. be embarrassed or resentful of the child,
        c. grieve or feel guilty,
        d. take on some degree of parental responsibility, or
        e. have trouble dealing with peer reactions.

    3. Grandparents may

        a. misunderstand or refuse to accept the diagnosis,
        b. feel grief or guilt, or
        c. support family members.

D. Challenges after diagnosis

    1. Emotional challenges

        a. Family relationships: conflict among needs of individual members.
        b. Family changes: members having to assume different roles.
        c. Coping emotionally: coming to terms with having a child with a disability.
        d. Living with worry and anxiety: uncertainty about the child's long-term outcome.
        e. Hospital experiences and relationships with professionals: fear and resentment of staff's power over the child or themselves.
        f. Finding meaning: making sense of the situation.
        g. Dealing with social shame and isolation: how to share information and feelings with others.

      h.   Parents' reproductive decisions: fear of having another child with special needs; child's caretaking needs interfering with planning future pregnancies.

  2.   Task-oriented challenges

      a.   Learning about the child's condition: having to master complex information and learn new procedures rapidly while coping with the child's diagnosis.

      b.   Accessing services: assessing the child's and family's needs; learning about services and getting services; balancing needs for many services from many places.

      c.   Financial concerns: costs of treatment and care; renegotiating what insurance covers and what may not be necessary. The child's illnesses or crises may interfere with a parent's ability to work full time, reliably, or at all.

III. Factors affecting how families cope

  A.   Family functioning

    1.   To recover from adversity and adjust to change, families have to:

      a.   Balance the illness or disability with other family needs.

          (1)   Balance the child's special needs with his/her other developmental needs.

          (2)   Balance the child's needs with other family members' needs.

          (3)   Make an effort to maintain the family's routine and identity.

      b.   Maintain clear boundaries and retain control of the family's needs and preferences.

      c.   Communicate feelings, thoughts, and concerns.

      d.   See something positive in the situation or find new meaning in life.

      e.   Maintain family flexibility.

          (1)   "Shift gears" and adapt to changing circumstances.

          (2)   Don't allow rigid compliance to meet the needs of the child with special needs to

be achieved at the expense of brothers, sisters, and family development.

    (3)   Be flexible in setting rules, establishing roles, and defining expectations.

f.   Maintain a commitment to the family unit and to keeping the family together.

g.   Engage in active coping efforts.

    (1)   Seek information about the disability.
    (2)   Find needed services for the child.
    (3)   Achieve a sense of mastery that allows the family to maintain its honor and independence.

h.   Anticipate the family's needs and actively seek information and support.

i.   Develop good working relationships with professionals.

2.   Less adaptive families may not function as well or may not stay together.

B.   Characteristics of the child with special needs

    1.   Temperament

    2.   Sex

    3.   Ordinal position in the family (birth order)

    4.   Age

    5.   Attractiveness

C.   Nature of the disability or chronic condition

    1.   How extensive and noticeable the disability is

    2.   How demanding the child's care is

    3.   How society reacts to the disability or condition

D.   The community

    1.   Formal networks

        a.   health, mental health, and social services
        b.   child care

        c. early intervention programs
        d. educational systems

   2. Informal networks

        a. neighbors, friends, co-workers
        b. churches and religious groups
        c. other parents who have children with disabilities

IV. Family-centered care: An intervention philosophy

   A. Principles underlying family-centered care

      1. The family is a constant in the child's life; intervention settings are temporary.

      2. The family determines its needs and priorities and makes all decisions, including the right to refuse or postpone services.

      3. Individual differences between families must be respected.

        a. Families have different strengths and patterns of coping with problems.
        b. Cultural differences must be respected.

   B. Factors to consider when providing family-centered services

      1. Some families refuse outside help.

      2. Some families feel isolated from information or services.

      3. A family's values and cultural perspective may differ from those of service providers.

      4. Individual family members may react differently to a child with special needs and to service providers.

   C. Strategies for effective partnerships between caregivers and parents

      1. Listen to what the family identifies as the needs of the child and family.

      2. Accept the family, not just the child, as the focus of services.

3. Try to understand how the family functions and how its members function within the family.

4. Support the family's decisions concerning care and interventions for their child.

5. Share information and resources, and help with referrals for services.

6. Share information on the child's development and behavior in a supportive way. Provide feedback about the child's strengths and progress. Encourage parents to think in "small steps."

7. Individualize your approach to each child and family. Be flexible and responsive to the unique needs of different families and children.

8. When imparting or requesting information, consider all family members.

9. Encourage both parents to attend conferences and school activities.

10. Prepare families for changes in the child-care setting (for example, transitions from the toddler room to preschool).

11. Encourage parents to support other parents who have children with special needs.

12. Encourage families to seek and use help from various sources.

13. Encourage families to become aware of their legal rights and options, such as the right to an IFSP (individual family service plan).

BIBLIOGRAPHY

Brown, W., Thurman, S. K., & Pearl, L. F. (1993). *Family-centered early intervention with infants and toddlers: Innovative cross-disciplinary approaches.* Baltimore: Paul H. Brookes Publishing.

Costello, A. (1988). The psychological impact of genetic disease. In *Genetic applications: A health perspective.* Lawrence, KS: Learner Managed Designs.

Featherstone, H. (1980). *A difference in the family.* New York: Basic Books.

Leff, P. T., & Walizer, E. H. (1992). *Building the healing partnership: Parents, professionals and children with chronic illnesses and disabilities.* Cambridge, MA: Brookline Books.

McWilliam, P. J., & Bailey, D. B. (Eds.) (1993). *Working together with children and families: Case studies in early intervention.* Baltimore: Paul H. Brookes.

Singer, G. H. S., & Powers, L.E. (Eds.). (1993). *Families, disabilities and empowerment: Active coping skills and strategies for family interventions.* Baltimore: Paul H. Brookes.

Turnbull, A., & Turnbull, H. (1986). *Families, professionals, and exceptionality: A special partnership.* Columbus, OH: Merrill Publishing.

RESOURCES

Association for the Care of Children's Health, 7910 Woodmont Avenue, Suite 300, Bethesda, MD 20814-3015; (301) 654-6549

INCLUSION

I. Definitions

A. *Inclusion:* the full integration of children with disabilities into the same settings available to children without disabilities, in the same classroom for the entire day and in the same activities.

B. *Mainstreaming:* partial integration of children with disabilities into settings available to children without disabilities. Generally, children with disabilities are in some classes separate from the other children and are included in general education classrooms for part of the day.

C. *Segregation:* the separation of children with disabilities from children without disabilities; children with disabilities attend special education classes and do not mingle with other children.

D. *Least restrictive environment (LRE):* the concept, incorporated into law, that children with disabilities must be included in general education classrooms whenever possible. LRE originally was intended to decrease the number of children in institutional settings and segregated classrooms.

E. *Early intervention:* recognition, diagnosis, and treatment of developmental delay or potential delay in children birth to 5 years old. Based on the theory that the younger the child, and the less well established the delay, the greater the likelihood that the delay can be minimized or eliminated. Interventions include infant stimulation, therapy, family support and education, specialized health services, and coordination of services.

II. General principles

A. Inclusion is a commitment to children with disabilities. It is an attitude rather than just a behavior. It goes beyond the classroom and into the community. It holds that children with disabilities have the right to participate in activities that are open to children without disabilities — sports clubs, recreation center programs, cultural experiences, and so on.

B. Children with disabilities in inclusive settings are not expected to keep up with other children or to complete work that other children may complete. Rather, children with disabilities work at their own pace and at their own level. (Interactions between children with and without disabilities are supported.)

C. Inclusive settings for children with disabilities is not an entitlement; rather, federal regulations encourage these programs as a model for best practice.

D. Inclusion can be a parental choice. Not all parents wish to have their child in an inclusive setting. Once the benefits have been explained to the family, the final decision rests with the family.

III.   Federal legislation

A. Individuals with Disabilities Education Act (IDEA)

1. Established in 1991, IDEA was reauthorized in 1997.

2. Provides for a free, appropriate public education to all children with disabilities 3–21 years of age.

3. Requires that children with disabilities receive educational services in the Least Restrictive Environment.

4. Requires an individualized education program (IEP) for children with disabilities 3–21 years of age.

5. Places responsibility for identification of children with disabilities from birth to age 21 years on Child Identification or Child Find.

6. Is administered individually by each state's Department of Education (even though it is a federal law).

B. Part C of IDEA

1. Guides early intervention services for children birth to 3 years.

2. Directs each state to coordinate early intervention efforts among agencies and service providers and to identify children who qualify for early intervention services.

3. Defines the Individualized Family Service Plan (IFSP), which recognizes the interdependence of the young child and family and includes family support, the child's educational, therapeutic, and health needs.

Reference: OSERS (1997, June). Individuals with Disabilities Education Act Amendments of 1997. IDEA Home Page, US Department of Education Individuals with Disabilities Education Act Amendments of 1997, available at http://www.ed.gov/office/OSERS/IDEA/the_law.html

C. Americans with Disabilities Act (ADA)

1. Civil rights legislation enacted in 1991, prohibiting discrimination against people with disabilities.

   a. Applies to all commercial and public facilities, including child care centers, family day care homes, and preschools.
   b. Requires that all public facilities make "reasonable accommodations" to allow people with disabilities to use those facilities.

2. Defines an individual with a disability (child or adult) as one who

   a. ". . . has a physical or mental impairment which substantially limits one or more of the major life activities such as caring for oneself, performing manual tasks, walking, seeing, hearing, speaking, breathing, learning and working;
   b. has a record of such an impairment; or
   c. is regarded as having such an impairment."[1]

IV. **Implications for children with special needs**

A. Infants, toddlers, and preschoolers may not be denied entrance to a center simply because of a disability or chronic condition.

B. More children will have the opportunity to participate in a range of activities in their communities.

C. Children with disabilities and chronic conditions may receive therapeutic services within community child care and preschool settings.

D. Centers must be prepared to admit children with disabilities and chronic conditions.

---

[1] From *Child Care Settings and the Americans with Disabilities Act*, The Arc, 500 East Border Street, Third floor, Arlington, Texas 76010 (May, 1992)

V.   **Benefits of including young children with disabilities and chronic conditions in child care and preschools**

    A.   Children with and without disabilities develop an appreciation of each other and of individual differences.

    B.   When children with and without disabilities are integrated, acceptance and tolerance begin at an early age.

    C.   Inclusion expands the child's experiences and thereby facilitates learning.

    D.   Inclusion can promote social interaction between children with and without disabilities.

VI.   **Barriers to including young children with disabilities in child care and preschool**

    A.   Negative attitudes toward inclusion.

    B.   Lack of knowledge about young children with disabilities and chronic conditions.

    C.   Concerns that children without disabilities will be harmed physically, psychologically, or intellectually by their association with children who have disabilities.

    D.   Lack of resources and supports.

    E.   Physical barriers, such as no wheelchair ramps.

    F.   Concerns about health risks.

    G.   Concerns about possible costs required to make changes in the facility, staff, or policies.

VII.   **Strategies for inclusion in the child care setting**

    A.   When preparing for the admission of a child with a disability or chronic condition into the program:

        1.   Ask the child's parent/guardian about the child's abilities, likes, and dislikes.

        2.   Ask about treatments or therapies the parent/guardian is working on at home.

3. Ask about methods the parent/guardian has found helpful to stimulate the child and assist the child in learning.

4. Discuss specific needs and concerns the parent/ guardian has about inclusion.

5. Maintain confidentiality of medical and personal information.

B. Use "people first" language, focusing on the child rather than on the disability or illness (example: use "child with epilepsy" rather than "epileptic child").

C. Promote accessibility of the environment, not just barrier-free but also child-centered.

1. Be sure all children, regardless of mobility, can reach toys, tables, and easels.

2. Allow enough open space for children to move freely.

3. Check for smooth flooring between play areas.

4. Be sure potty chairs are easy to get to and adapted as needed.

5. Offer toys that are appropriate for the developmental level of all children, as well as toys adapted to a child's specific needs.

D. Encourage all children to join in activities.

1. Assist the child with a disability or chronic condition so that he/she may participate in activities.

2. Provide multisensory activities - those that involve speech, hearing, movement, touch, and sight.

3. Allow time for the child to get from place to place independently.

4. Allow choices and varied activities that are appropriate for the range of developmental levels of all children in the room.

5. Offer gentle verbal encouragement to participate, but do not force children to do so. Instead, provide a variety of interesting activities.

6.   Provide toys and activities that require interaction, such as music games, building blocks, water play.

7.   Model positive behaviors for young children, encouraging them to interact with the child with a disability or chronic condition.

E.   Make mealtime a shared activity.

1.   Be sure all children can reach chairs and table easily and that this furniture is secure.

2.   Have children who require special feeding techniques eat at the same table as the other children.

3.   As needed, make adaptations such as cut-out cups, built-up utensils, and plates that stay put.

F.   Treat all children with respect, dignity, and fairness.

1.   Keep in mind that children with disabilities are more *like* than unlike other children.

2.   Do not give special privileges to a child with a disability or chronic condition.

3.   Give all children warm support.

4.   Maintain the same standards of behavior for all children.

5.   Offer praise for achievements.

6.   Recognize each child's uniqueness.

BIBLIOGRAPHY

Abbott, C., & Gold, S. (1991). Conferring with parents when you're concerned that they need special services. *Young Children, 46,* 10-14.

ARC. *Child care settings and the Americans with Disabilities Act* (1992). Arlington, TX: ARC National Headquarters.

Delaney, N., & Zolondick, K. (1991). Day care for technology-dependent infants and young children: A new alternative. *Journal of Perinatal and Neonatal Nursing, 5*(1) 80-85.

Urbano, M. (1992). *Preschool children with special health care needs.* San Diego: Singular Publishing Group.

RESOURCES

The Arc, 500 East Border Street, Third floor, Arlington, TX 76010; (817) 261-6003

Educational Home Model Outreach Project, Rural Institute, University of Montana, 52 North Corbin Hall, Missoula, MT 59812

IMPLICATIONS OF POVERTY

I. Definitions

A. Poverty refers to the condition of living with insufficient economic resources.

    1. Poverty may affect people of all races, ethnic groups, and religions.

    2. Poverty implies both material hardship and experiences that other parts of society may not share, such as preoccupation with survival-related issues.

B. Poverty line

    1. The poverty line is a federally determined cash income level before taxes, adjusted for family size and changes in the cost of living, which is used to define poverty. Families whose incomes fall below the designated figure are considered "poor."

    2. The poverty line is used to determine eligibility for federal and state assistance programs.

    3. The poverty line is computed as three times the federal estimate of the cost of food for a family, but it underestimates the income needed to sustain a family.

    4. Low-income wage earners whose families are above the poverty line may not be eligible for many assistance programs; often referred to as the "working poor."

II. Causes of poverty in families with young children

A. "The prime cause of poverty in American families is the financial abandonment of children, mostly by absent fathers."[1]

B. Shifts away from well-paid manufacturing jobs to more jobs in lower-paying service industries (for example, fast food restaurants) also contribute to poverty in families.

---

[1] From *From Cradle to Grave: The Human Face of Poverty in America*, by J. Freedman (New York: Athencum, 1993), p. 135.

III.   **Incidence of poverty among children and related statistics.**[2]
        The number of children living in poverty is increasing.

   A.   In 1993, 25.6%, or about 6 million, of U.S. children under
         age 6 were living in poverty.

   B.   In 1993, the poverty line for a family of three was well
         above the annual salary of a minimum wage job.

      1.   More than 60% of children living in poverty were in
            households where someone was employed.

      2.   More than 20% of children living in poverty were in
            households where someone was employed year
            round, full time.

   C.   The likelihood that a family lives in poverty
         rises with the following factors:

      1.   Child poverty is concentrated among ethnic and racial
            minorities.

      2.   Households headed by women are far more likely to
            be poor.

      3.   As family size increases, the risk of poverty
            increases.

   D.   1992 census data provided the following distribution of
         poverty among children under age 6:[3]

      1.   35% of children in urban areas lived in poverty.

      2.   19% of children in suburban areas lived in poverty.

      3.   28% of children in rural areas lived in poverty.

---

[2] From *The State of America's Children Yearbook: 1995,* by the Children's Defense
     Fund (Washington, DC: Children's Defense Fund, 1995).

[3] From "Number of Poor Children Under Six Increased from 5 to 6 Million 1987-
     1992," by National Center for Children in Poverty, *News and Issues (Columbia
     University School of Public Health),* 5(1) (Winter/Spring, 1995).

IV. **Impact of living in poverty.** Poverty increases the risk for the factors listed below but does not ensure them.

    A. Pregnant women living in poverty are more likely to

        1. have a poor health history before becoming pregnant,

        2. lack adequate prenatal care and nutrition,

        3. undergo significant stress during pregnancy,

        4. be at increased risk for use of drugs and alcohol,

        5. be exposed to HIV, and

        6. deliver prematurely and deliver children with poor birth outcomes.

    B. Children living in poverty are likely to have

        1. inadequate diet (for example, fruit drink mixes instead of juice); especially lacking in iron intake;

        2. inadequate medical and dental care, particularly immunizations and other preventive measures;

        3. toxic blood levels (from exposure to environmental toxins such as lead);

        4. higher incidence of injury and health problems, including asthma, fractures, pneumonia, poisoning, and recurrent ear infection; and

        5. more frequent hospitalizations with longer stays.

    C. Families living in poverty have fewer choices.

        1. Residential choices are more limited. Children may be exposed to

            a. unsafe neighborhoods — crime and violence in the neighborhood;

            b. inadequate and unsafe housing — homelessness, poor neighborhood sanitation, home that is not "child-proof," lead-based paint, nonworking appliances, inadequate plumbing and heat/air, broken or unsafe windows, poor or no home maintenance;

    c.   overcrowding;

    d.   residential instability — frequent moves result-
ing in difficulty qualifying for local services;
disruption of services, routines, and bonding
with caregivers; and

    e.   homelessness — an estimated 10% of families
with young children are homeless.[4]

2.   The quality of the schools attended may be low, and
the likelihood of graduating from high school is
lower.

3.   Subsidized rates paid for children with low family
incomes may not attract top-quality providers, leading
to higher likelihood of inadequate child care.

4.   Children may be at higher risk of injury or disability
because of

    a.   inadequate safety precautions and supervision,

    b.   exposure to violence, and

    c.   exposure to lead.

5.   Day-to-day choices are more limited. Inadequate
income is accompanied by fewer changes of clothes
and diapers, "extras" such as field trips and school
supplies create a financial burden, and local services
are chosen over more distant (and possibly better)
ones when transportation is inadequate.

6.   People with low income spend more time waiting for
buses, doctors, appointments, and the like.

7.   In chronic poverty conditions, irregular or erratic
waking, sleeping, and meal schedules, irregular
places to sleep, and fluctuation in household
composition are common.

---

[4] From "Poverty and Infant Development," by R. Halpern, in *Handbook of Infant Mental Health*, edited by C. H. Zeanah (New York: Guilford Press, 1993), p. 76.

D. The nature of rural poverty

   1. Rural areas typically have especially high numbers of

      a. children living in poverty,
      b. migrants,
      c. non-English speaking people, and
      d. minorities.

   2. In addition to poverty, rural areas often are characterized by

      a. isolation (by definition),
      b. high unemployment,
      c. ready availability of weapons,
      d. little public transportation, and
      e. inadequate health service accessibility.

E. The continuing emotional stress of never having enough money may undermine parenting by

   1. contributing to a sense of powerlessness or inadequacy as a parent,

   2. magnifying preexisting parental risk factors (such as an inborn risk of depression), and

   3. focusing concern on a child's material well-being at the expense of emotional well-being.

V. Implications for children with special needs

A. Threat to the family structure[5]

   1. 80% of marriages fail when a very sick child is born.

   2. Parents go through severe emotional, personal, and financial stresses that may weaken their relationship, increasing the likelihood that the child will be reared in a single-parent family.

   3. If the family lacks resources to pay the costs of health care for a child with special needs, caseworkers may encourage divorce to make the child eligible for Medicaid.

---

[5] From *From Cradle to Grave: The Human Face of Poverty in America,* by J. Freedman (New York: Atheneum, 1993).

B.   Prenatal risk factors

1.   Fetal alcohol syndrome and prenatal substance exposure.

2.   Pediatric AIDS and other prenatal infections.

3.   Intrauterine growth retardation; small for gestational age.

4.   Prematurity.

C.   Lifestyle issues

1.   Children with special health care needs require more frequent and more costly health and medical care.

2.   Many children with a disability or chronic condition need more time and more parental patience in accomplishing routine tasks. If the parent is under chronic stress because of living in poverty, meeting the daily child's needs may be difficult.

3.   Frequent moves or disruptions in services make continuous relationships with caregivers less likely for those living in poverty.   Disruptions in caregiving, if coupled with parenting problems, can be particularly hard on children with special needs.

4.   The need for frequent travel to health and therapy appointments is complicated if a family lacks good transportation, particularly for a child in a wheelchair or requiring equipment.

5.   Children with special needs living in rural areas have less access to services, especially specialists and special facilities. For example, in a health crisis, the nearest hospital may be hours away. If a family cannot afford a reliable vehicle, the consequences become worse.

VI. **Resources for children and families living in poverty**

    A. Federal resources

        1. *Early and Periodic Screening, Diagnosis and Treatment Program (EPSDT)* for children, birth through 21 years, provides all medically necessary services, including diagnosis, to

            a. maintain functioning level;
            b. prevent further decline of developmental or health status; and/or
            c. improve the health status of children when possible.

        2. *Title V* funding for services to children with disabilities for families living below the poverty line, and (with fees on a sliding scale) to those living up to 185% of the poverty line.

            a. These programs usually are administered through the state health department.
            b. They may be referred to as "programs for children with special health care needs" or "programs for children with disabilities."

        3. *Public education.* For children with disabilities age 3 years and older, the public school system must provide a free and appropriate public education. This may include health services necessary for the child to benefit from the education. This includes Child Find services to identify and serve children with disabilities from birth through 5 years of age.

        4. *Head Start.* This program serves children living in low-income areas. At least 10% of all enrollment is reserved for children with disabilities or developmental delays.

    B. State and local resources

        1. Early intervention centers provide assessment, intervention, referral, and case management services.

        2. Home-based services, provided by public and private service agencies in the child's home.

        3. Medical centers provide access to health professionals and facilitate referrals for special services.

4. Service clubs such as the Lions, Kiwanas, and Elks — may provide limited funding for services or medical equipment on an individual basis.

5. Religious groups and churches — may provide limited funding for services such as respite care.

6. Support groups or information associations for specific disorders or disabilities — may provide services or referral for children with specified disabilities.

7. Insurance companies or health maintenance organizations — services may have to be preapproved or provided by an approved service provider.

BIBLIOGRAPHY

Children's Defense Fund (1995). *The state of America's children yearbook: 1995.* Washington, DC: CDF.

Freedman, J. (1993). *From cradle to grave: The human face of poverty in America.* New York: Atheneum.

Halpern, R. (1993). Poverty and infant development. In C. H. Zeanah (Ed.), *Handbook of infant mental health,* 73-86. New York: Guilford Press.

Thompson, T. & Hupp, S. C. (Eds.) (1992). *Saving children at risk: Poverty and disabilities.* Newbury Park, CA: Sage.

LEGAL ISSUES

I. Liability issues

A. Definitions

1. *Negligence:* the omission or neglect of reasonable precaution, care, or action.

2. *Duty:* the obligation to act toward another as a reasonably prudent person would under the circumstances.

3. *Breach:* failing to act toward another as a reasonably prudent person would under the circumstances.

4. *Liability:* the responsibility one bears for the breach of a duty.

B. Areas for concern/risk

1. Transportation (special requirements/needs/equipment)

2. Administration of medications[1]

3. Noncompliance with State or County regulations

4. Poor hygiene procedures

5. Failure to obtain necessary licenses/inspections

6. Inadequate/improper training of staff

7. Inadequate supervision of staff

8. Lack of documentation (written procedures)

---

[1] Administration of medication is generally regarded as an invasive procedure and, as such, is a nursing task that may be subject to statutory provisions or to regulations established by your State's Nursing Board. If this is the case, legislation or regulatory guidelines may be in place that determine whether or not and how this task may be delegated to a non-health-licensed individual (other than the child's parent or guardian). For the safety of the children, and due to the risk of personal and agency liability, you are urged to contact your State Board of Nursing to inquire about the status of delegation of invasive procedures in your state.

9.   Lack of written health care plan for individual child

10. Hiring individual without conducting background check, particularly for any history of abuse

11. Breach of confidentiality

II.   Business details (written policies and procedures)

A.   Determining incorporation, nonprofit status, corporate status, and the like

B.   Written policies regarding acceptance of ill children, isolation of ill children, trial period,[2] discipline procedures, payment during child's absences, notice requirements for termination by center or parent/guardian, nonpayment/ disenrollment procedures, confidentiality

C.   Written release of information for health care professionals (physicians, nurses, physical therapists, occupational therapists, as required)

D.   Written meal plans/menus (may be on rotating calendar) to alert caregivers to potential food allergy issues

E.   Written arrangement for physician/nursing services or consultation to center

F.   Written procedures for

1.   administration of medication[3] that complies with State or County regulations, and State Nurse Practice Act;

2.   hygiene procedures (handwashing, bodily fluids, hazardous waste, infant care versus toddler and older); and/or

---

[2] A trial period is a probation period to see if the child and the center are a good "match" and the center can meet the child's needs while meeting the needs of the other children.

[3] See footnote 1.

    3. knowledge and documentation of insurance coverage policies:

       a. commercial liability,
       b. homeowners or center liability policy, and
       c. automobile policy coverage maximums.

G. Written agreements used as waivers of liability with reference to

    1. transportation by center personnel, and

    2. agreements regarding provision of health services to child by private health care professionals on the center premises,

H. Written health care plan:

    1. for every child requiring one,

    2. to include procedures and personnel needed to carry out procedures, and

    3. to include policies regarding resuscitation of child to be provided to all staff members.

III. Communication between parents/guardians and staff

A. At least one staff person should be designated to resolve parent/guardian complaints.

B. A system should be developed for communicating regularly with parents/guardians.

    1. Mailboxes can be placed at the center and parents/guardians asked to check them.

    2. Back-and-forth folder system might be used.

    3. Some parents/guardians need daily communication and some need only weekly communication.

    4. Policies should be set regarding telephoning staff at home or after hours as well as a time frame (such as 24 hours) for staff to respond to parents.

IV.   Compliance with Americans with Disabilities Act (ADA)

A.   Accessibility to the center for parents/guardians.

B.   Nondiscrimination policies regarding enrollment.

C.   Ability to identify and meet children's special needs.

D.   Accommodations that are financially reasonable given the center's budget.

V.   Compliance with Section 504 of Rehabilitation Act of 1973

A.   If any federal monies are received, the child care center must comply with equal opportunity and nondiscriminatory policies of this federal statute. These monies may be received as grants, flow-through funds, and so on.

B.   A person with a disability is defined here as one who has an impairment that affects his/her ability to see, hear, walk, talk, breathe, learn, or work.

C.   The center must comply as to both staff and children.

RESOURCES

American Bar Association, Center on Children & the Law, 1800 M Street NW, Suite S-200, Washington, DC 20036; (202) 662-1720

Children's Defense Fund, 25 E Street NW, Washington, DC 20001; (202) 628-8787

State Protection and Advocacy Agency: Contact National Protection and Advocacy System, Washington, DC; (202) 408-9514

Faculty members of state universities with an education department

RESPECTING DIVERSITY

I. **Definition:** For purposes of this lesson, *diversity* refers to differences among people — differences in ethnicity, culture, religion, language, socioeconomic status, and presence or absence of a disability or chronic condition.

II. **General principles**

    A. Expanded awareness and knowledge of people with diverse backgrounds increases learning and may improve competence in providing care for children who are different from oneself.

    B. Helping children learn to value diversity may build positive perceptions, beliefs, and behaviors toward people who are different.

    C. Valuing diversity and appreciating differences help to eliminate negative stereotyping.

    D. Settings with diverse groups of people offer an opportunity to learn about and benefit from other people's cultural and personal attributes.

    E. Respecting diversity means learning about similarities as well as differences between and among families.

    F. Great diversity is found even within cultural groups. Therefore, no hard-and-fast rules can be offered about relating to individuals from other ethnic and cultural backgrounds. To extend the most effective child care services, caregivers must appreciate and respond to *individual differences*.

III. **Culture and disability as elements of diversity**

    A. Communication

        1. Families differ in communication styles and methods.

        2. Families may use different languages to communicate, and they may or may not be bilingual.

        3. Individuals differ in the ways they speak, such as the pace of speech or accents in their speech.

        4. People from different cultures differ in the physical distance they prefer in various types of interactions.

5. The use of touch in communication means different things to people of different cultures. In one cultural context, touching a child on the head may be a gesture of admiration; in another, it may be construed as placing a curse on the child.

6. Gestures and body language may be an important part of communication. For example, direct eye contact is a sign of disrespect or a sign of attentiveness depending upon one's culture.

7. Families of children with hearing loss differ in their preferences regarding American Sign Language, lipreading, or other methods of communication.

8. Children who are unable to talk because of a disability might use a communication device such as a pointer board, a touch talker, or Liberator™ (a complex electronic communication device).

9. Families who speak in a language other than English are entitled to an interpreter when discussing matters that affect the health, safety, or well-being of their child.

B. Physical differences

1. People differ in color of skin, hair, and eyes.

2. "Normal" height and weight ratios for age vary by ethnic background.

3. Height and weight differences may be influenced both by culture and by disability. For example, a child of Filipino background may be smaller in size because of ethnic heritage as well as effects of a congenital heart defect.

4. Children with disabilities come from every cultural background.

5. Certain disabilities or chronic health conditions are more common in individuals of specific ethnic heritage. Examples are the greater prevalence of spina bifida in children of Irish-English background; sickle cell disease in children of African-American background; and lactose (a component of milk) intolerance, more common in individuals from Asian cultures.

C. Family relationships

    1.   The family structure and roles/responsibilities of family members vary according to their cultural heritage. For example, Haitian families in general value the mother as a stabilizing influence; her influence extends into the child's adulthood, even to areas of marriage and job choice.

    2.   The wife may be expected to stay home and take care of the house and children while the husband works, or parents may share equally in work and child care.

    3.   Families may be large or small, and extended family members such as grandparents, aunts and uncles, or cousins may live in the home; or a family may include unrelated adults and children. Extended families are more important in some cultures than others.

    4.   Decision making about family matters may rest with the father or the mother, with an elder relation, or may be shared by both parents.

    5.   Family structure and distribution of responsibilities may influence who provides the day-to-day care of a child with a disability or chronic condition, as well as who makes the decisions regarding child care, school, and health care.

D. Child-rearing practices

    1.   Attitudes toward children's behavior and discipline are determined by cultural background, habits of the parents' families, and the parents' experiences. Children with disabilities may be allowed more, or less, latitude in behavior than children without disabilities.

    2.   Great cultural differences are found in the types of behavior considered acceptable. For example, children from traditional Japanese backgrounds are expected to be quiet, respectful, and obedient to their elders at all times.

    3.   In most cultures the primary caregiver is the mother. In others, however, it may be the grandmother or an aunt. In some cultures godparents are expected to help the family provide for the child's welfare.

4. Children in some cultures are expected to contribute to the family welfare at an early age — by dropping out of school to work, for example.

5. Families differ in their beliefs about the timing and method of potty training. For example, Hmong families (from Southeast Asia) expect children to train themselves.

6. Attitudes toward children with disabilities and chronic conditions also are affected by culture. In some Asian and Hispanic cultures, a child with a disability is seen as blessed, conferring good will upon the family.

E. Health care

1. Families differ in their perceptions of health and illness, as well as in the treatment of illness.

2. Some cultures hold that illness is caused by an imbalance of energy within the body. Some believe that illness is caused by supernatural forces or actions of the child's parents or ancestors.

3. Many cultures use folk or traditional treatments to treat common ailments. Traditional Vietnamese families may treat minor illnesses in children with "coining," or rubbing a coin over the surface of the skin, causing discoloration; or "cupping," applying suction to a cup or glass placed on the skin, causing a bruise. Marks left on the skin by this traditional healing method may be mistaken for child abuse.

4. Families of children with disabilities or chronic conditions may subscribe to traditional, culturally based methods or to Western scientific medicine, or both approaches.

F. Cultural considerations

1. The term *cultural norms* refers to accepted behavior regarding expression of emotions or feelings, religion, and response to illness, disability, and death.

2.   Culture or religious background affects a family's willingness to talk about problems with a stranger or an acquaintance, such as a caregiver. A child's behavior at home or the steps a family is taking to address a child's illness may be regarded as private matters not to be shared.

3.   Culture may influence time orientations, resulting in situations such as a parent showing up chronically late to pick up a child or arriving early or late for a meeting with caregivers. Differences in time orientation also may become frustrating for family and caregiver alike when planning ahead for services or when providing interventions focused on long-term changes.

G.   Diet and nutritional preferences

1.   Food preferences of families may be influenced both by ethnic heritage and by beliefs about the healing or healthful properties of foods.

2.   Families of certain Asian backgrounds believe that foods have either hot or cold properties (distinct from the foods' actual temperature) that may cure illness or keep an individual healthy.

3.   Some families are vegetarian, based on their beliefs about health, the environment, or religion.

4.   Ethnic food preferences and food preparation habits may differ from medical recommendations and complicate the care of children with disabilities. For example, high-fat, high-protein meals can increase the risk of obesity in many children with disabilities such as Down syndrome and spina bifida.

H.   Religion

1.   Religious beliefs may influence health care choices, as well as how the family chooses to care for a child with a disability. For instance, instead of using a physician, Christian Scientists seek the assistance of a Christian Scientist Reader during times of illness.

2. Families may insist that their child wear certain religious articles. As examples, many Catholics wear religious medals depicting saints, and Laotian children may wear cloth or leather bracelets meant to protect them from illness or evil spirits.

3. Families observe different holidays, serve special holiday foods, or fast (choose not to eat or drink anything) during holidays. Jewish people fast on Yom Kippur. Muslim families fast from sunrise to sunset during Ramadan (usually, children participate in these fasts in a modified way or only upon maturity).

IV. Differential treatment of children with disabilities

A. Throughout history, children with disabilities or chronic conditions have been singled out and treated differently from their peers. Some reasons for differential treatment are

1. care of the child interfered with the group's survival,

2. any child who differed significantly from the ideal was not valued, and

3. supernatural or negative qualities were attributed to the child.

B. Differential treatment persists today; children with a disability or chronic condition may be

1. shunned socially,
2. isolated for special care,
3. feared as having a contagious condition, or
4. perceived as less deserving than other children or as unaware that they are being treated differently.

V. Implications for caregivers of young children with disabilities and their families

A. Breaking down barriers for children with disabilities

1. Listen to parents, children, siblings, and peers who have lifestyles different from ours.

2. When circumstances indicate, seek advice/counsel from people of other cultures, backgrounds, abilities/disabilities. Take into account individual and cultural considerations (keeping in mind that people may or may not have been reared in customs traditional to their culture).

3. Learn about other cultures, lifestyles, and abilities/disabilities, keeping in mind that there is no one answer or recipe for working with children with disabilities or children from diverse backgrounds.

4. Talk with adults or older children with disabilities about their experiences growing up with a disability.

5. Through reading, movies, and literature, learn about how other cultures view disabilities.

B. In examining your current beliefs, ask yourself:

1. What values/beliefs/assumptions are most important to you (family, career, spiritual life, and so on)?

2. Would you be willing to exchange your values with those of the person sitting next to you (for example, your religious beliefs)?

3. How do your actions/behaviors represent your beliefs?

4. What are your beliefs and feelings about children who have disabilities?

5. How do families with backgrounds different from yours (generational, ethnic, cultural, disabilities) respond to you, and how do you respond to them?

6. What attitudes or assumptions do you hold about specific groups (such as children with disabilities, different socioeconomic status)?

7. How do you convey your feelings and attitudes (consciously/unconsciously) to people who are different from you?

VI. **Incorporating diversity in the child care setting**

A. Decorate rooms with posters and photos that depict people, including children, from diverse backgrounds.

   1. Use books and pictures that depict children with and without disabilities.

   2. Provide dolls and materials that represent children from diverse backgrounds with and without disabilities in both traditional and modern dress.

   3. Provide hands-on diversity materials (musical instruments, clothing).

   4. Offer children the opportunity to try out adaptive equipment (crutches, augmentative communication, and so on).

   5. Make all items accessible to children throughout the year, not just within certain months or during holidays.

B. Invite people with disabilities and from different cultural and ethnic backgrounds to visit your setting (not just on holidays or certain months).

C. Talk without labeling. Use "people-first" language. For example, the term *disabled child* emphasizes the disability, whereas the term *child with a disability* puts the child first.

D. Speak positively about all children and people (avoid labeling and stereotyping).

BIBLIOGRAPHY

Abbott, C. & Gold, S. (1991). Conferring with parents when you're concerned that they need special services. *Young Children, 46,* 10-14.

Coleman, L. (1991). Planning for the changing nature of family life in schools for young children. *Young Children, 46,* 15-20.

Cook, R. E., Tessier, A., & Klein, M. D. (1992). *Adapting early childhood curricula for children with special needs.* New York: Merrill.

Ford, B., & Jones, C. (1990). Ethnic feelings book. *Teaching Exceptional Children, 22*(4), 36-39.

Gonzalez-Mena, J. (1992). Taking a culturally sensitive approach in infant-toddler programs. *Young Children, 47*(2), 12-18.

Groce, N., & Zola, K. (1993). Multiculturalism, chronic illness, and disability. *Pediatrics, 91*(5), (Supplement), 1048-1045.

Harris, C. (1991). Identifying and serving the gifted new immigrant: Problems and strategies. *Teaching Exceptional Children, 23*(4), 26-30.

Harry, B. (1992). Making sense of disability: Low-income, Puerto Rican parents' theories of the problem. *Exceptional Children, 59*(1), 27-40.

Harry, B., Allen, N., & McLaughlin, M. (1995). Communication versus compliance: African-American parents' involvement in special education. *Exceptional Children, 61*(2), 364-377.

Hyun, J., & Fowler, S. (1995). Respect, cultural sensitivity and communication: Promoting participation by Asian families in the individualized family service plan. *Teaching Exceptional Children, 28*(1), 23-28.

Klein, H. (1995). Urban Appalachian children in northern schools: A study in diversity. *Young Children, 50*(1), 10-73.

Klopf, D. W. (1991). *Intercultural encounters,* Englewood, CO: Morton Publishing.

Lynch, E., & Hanson, M. (1992). *Developing cross-cultural competence: A guide for working with young children and their families*. Baltimore: Paul H. Brookes.

Mallory, B., & New, R. (1994). *Diversity and developmentally appropriate practices*. New York: Teachers College Press.

McCracken Brown, J. (1993). *Valuing diversity: The primary years.* Washington, DC: National Association for the Education of Young Children.

McCubbin, H., Thompson, E., Thompson, A., McCubbin, M., & Kaston, A. (1993). Culture, ethnicity, and the family: Critical factors in childhood chronic illness and disabilities. *Pediatrics, 91*(5) (Supplement), 1063-1070.

Paterson, J., & Blum, R. (1993). A conference on culture and chronic illness in childhood: Conference summary. *Pediatrics, 91*(5) (Supplement), 1025-1030.

Peck, C. A., Odom, S. L., & Bricker, D. D. (1993). *Integrating young children with disabilities into community programs: Ecological perspectives on research and implementation.* Baltimore: Paul H. Brookes.

Randall-David, E. (1989). *Strategies for working with culturally diverse communities and clients.* Washington, DC: Association for the Care of Children's Health.

Schrefer, S. (Ed.). (1994). *Quick reference to cultural assessment.* St. Louis: Mosby-Year Book.

Seefeldt, C. (1993). Social studies: Learning for freedom. *Young Children, 48*(3), 4-16.

Shea, M. A. (1993). *On diversity in teaching and learning.* Boulder: University of Colorado.

"Teaching from a Multicultural Perspective." (1995). *CEC Today, 2*(2), 7 (published by Council for Exceptional Children).

RESOURCES

Association for the Care of Children's Health, 7910 Woodmont Avenue, Suite 300, Bethesda, MD 20814-3015; (301)-654-5649

Council for Exceptional Children, 1920 Association Drive, Reston, VA 22091-1589; (703) 620-3660

SUPPLEMENT: INVASIVE PROCEDURES

Medications

Clean Intermittent Catheterization (CIC)

Oxygen Therapy

Tracheostomy Care

Gastrostomy Care

MEDICATIONS

Objectives

- Recognize the responsibilities of the caregiver/preschool or center in giving medications.
- Recognize the basic principles for safe administration of medications.

I. Administration

 A. Administration of medication is considered an invasive procedure.

 B. The person who administers medication should receive instruction and supervision from a licensed health care provider according to state rules and regulations.

II. Responsibilities of parent/guardian

 A. Bring the medication request form, written instructions, prescription.

 B. Bring an adequate amount of the medication with information including

  1. date,

  2. child's name,

  3. dosage/amount to be given,

  4. reason for needing the medication,

  5. amount in bottle,

  6. method of administration,

  7. time(s) to be given,

  8. suggestions for giving the medication,

  9. side effects to watch for,

  10. need for refrigeration, and

  11. signature of parent/guardian.

III. Responsibilities of the caregiver

A.   Provide medication forms for parent/guardian.

B.   *Do not* accept medication unless it is in a prescription container for the designated child.

C.   Store medications in a locked cupboard or, if refrigeration is required, in a separate place in the refrigerator.

D.   Give medications at prescribed times.

E.   Report any difficulties with the child to the parent/guardian.

F.   Do not give any medication, including over-the-counter medications, without written authorization from physician.

G.   Whenever you give a medicine, record it on the child's medication record (date, time, dosage, caregiver's name).

IV. Giving medications

A.   Wash hands.

B.   Review the "five Rs:"

   1.   *R*ight child

   2.   *R*ight medication

   3.   *R*ight dose

   4.   *R*ight time

   5.   *R*ight route

BIBLIOGRAPHY

Graff, J. C. (1990). *Health care for students with disabilities; An illustrated medical guide for the classroom,* (Ch. 3: Medication administration). Baltimore: Paul H. Brookes.

Schmidt, B. (1991). *Your child's health: The parent's guide to symptoms, emergencies, common illnesses, behavior, and school problems* (rev. ed.). New York: Bantam Books.

CLEAN INTERMITTENT CATHETERIZATION (CIC)

Objectives:

- Be able to identify benefits of clean intermittent catheterization.
- Be acquainted with basic anatomy of the urinary tract.
- List special considerations with a child requiring clean intermittent catheterization.

I.   **What is clean intermittent catheterization**

    A.   *Clean intermittent catheterization (CIC):*   procedure in which a clean rubber or plastic catheter is inserted into the urethra and up into the bladder five or six times a day, using a clean, nonsterile technique, to release urine and empty the bladder.

    B.   Clean intermittent catheterization is an invasive procedure and must be performed by a specially trained individual who is supervised by a Registered Nurse or other licensed health care provider in accordance with state rules and regulations.

    C.   Common conditions requiring CIC include spina bifida and spinal cord injury.

II.   **Urinary system**

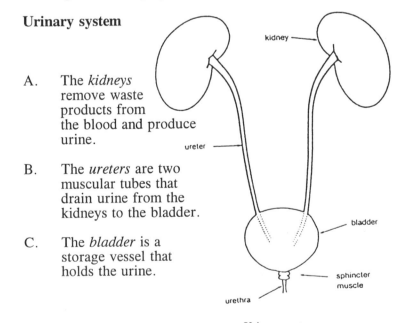

    A.   The *kidneys* remove waste products from the blood and produce urine.

    B.   The *ureters* are two muscular tubes that drain urine from the kidneys to the bladder.

    C.   The *bladder* is a storage vessel that holds the urine.

Urinary system

D.   The *urethra* is a muscular tube through which urine flows from the bladder out of the body.

E.   The *sphincter* is a circular muscle that opens and closes the urethra. When it closes, it stops the flow of urine out of the body.

III.   Benefits of clean intermittent catheterization

A.   Permits elimination of urine from the body.

B.   Helps to prevent bladder infections.

C.   Allows the child to stay dry and most like normal.

IV.   Requirements for clean intermittent catheterization

A.   In most states a prescription is required from the child's physician before catheterization can be performed in a child care or school setting.

B.   As with any invasive procedure, the individual who performs the catheterization in the child care or school setting must receive thorough instruction and supervision from a licensed health care provider.

C.   The child's parent/guardian usually provides the equipment and supplies needed to perform clean intermittent catheterization.

D.   Privacy should be provided to preschoolers and older children who require clean intermittent catheterization.

E.   Children with spina bifida often develop an allergy to latex products, so catheters and gloves should be non-latex.

F.   Caregivers should recognize the problems that can occur with clean intermittent catheterization and the person to contact if a problem occurs.

G.   Children with spina bifida and spinal cord injury are more likely than others to get bladder infections.

H.   Each child who requires clean intermittent catheterization should have a health care plan that describes the specific procedure and what to do when a problem occurs.

V.   Medications[1]

A.   The child's physician or specialist may prescribe medication to help improve bladder function.

B.   The caregiver should understand the desired effects of the medication as well as undesirable side effects.

BIBLIOGRAPHY

Graff, J. C. et al. (1990). *Health care for students with disabilities: An illustrated medical guide for the classroom.* Baltimore: Paul H. Brookes Publishing.

Smith, K. (1990). Bowel and bladder management of the child with myelomeningocele in the school setting. *Journal of Pediatric Care, 4*(4), 175-180.

Swinyard, C. A. *The child with spina bifida.* Chicago: Spina Bifida Association of America.

RESOURCES

Spina Bifida Association of America, 4590 MacArthur Blvd. NW, Suite 250, Washington, DC 20007-4226; (202) 944-3285, 1-800-621-3141

---

[1] Administration of medication is generally regarded as an invasive procedure and, as such, is a nursing task that may be subject to statutory provisions or to regulations established by your State's Nursing Board. If this is the case, legislation or regulatory guidelines may be in place that determine whether or not and how this task may be delegated to a non-health-licensed individual (other than the child's parent or guardian). For the safety of the children, and due to the risk of personal and agency liability, you are urged to contact your State Board of Nursing to inquire about the status of delegation of invasive procedures in your state.

OXYGEN THERAPY

Objectives:

- Identify special care needs of children who are dependent on oxygen
- Identify safety precautions to be taken when working with oxygen-dependent children
- Recognize signs of oxygen deprivation in children.

I.   **What is oxygen?**

    A.   A tasteless, odorless gas that makes up 21% of the air we breathe

    B.   Process in the body

        1.   Oxygen is inhaled into the lungs.
        2.   The oxygen passes from the lungs to the blood.
        3.   Blood oxygenates vital organs and tissues.
        4.   Carbon dioxide is produced as a waste product, transported by blood to the lungs, and exhaled through the nose and mouth.

II. **Who may require oxygen therapy?**

    A.   Premature infants with lung disease usually caused by bronchopulmonary dysplasia (BPD) (damage to the airways often resulting from mechanical ventilation used to treat life-threatening respiratory illness).

    B.   Infants and young children with low resistance to infection who get pneumonia and need temporary oxygen therapy

C.   Children with cystic fibrosis

D.   Children with severe asthma

E.   Children with diseases of the heart or lungs

III.   Benefits of oxygen therapy

A.   Oxygen therapy enables the child to breathe better.

B.   Oxygen therapy enables more calories to be used for physical growth instead of the work of breathing.

C.   Children who use oxygen may go outside and participate in appropriate activities.

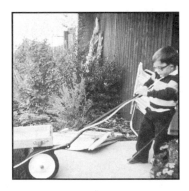

Child playing outside using portable oxygen supply

IV.   Legal considerations

A.   Oxygen therapy is an invasive procedure. The person who administers oxygen therapy must be a licensed health care professional, such as a nurse, or trained and supervised by a licensed health care professional.

B.   In most states a physician's prescription is required for oxygen administration in the child care or preschool setting.

V.   Oxygen delivery

A.   Two main types used are

1.   compressed gas
2.   liquid oxygen

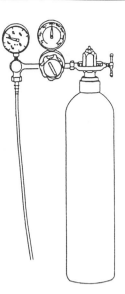

Portable tank for oxygen

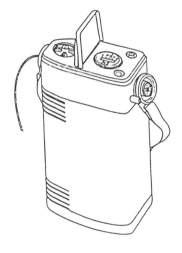

Portable tank for liquid oxygen

B.   Oxygen delivery devices may be portable or fixed.

C.   Variables in oxygen therapy include

1.   how long the oxygen will last,

2.   method for measuring the amount of oxygen the child receives,

3.   mechanisms to tell when the oxygen tank is full or is running out, and

4.   the company that supplies the oxygen.

D.   Nasal cannula delivers oxygen into the nose.

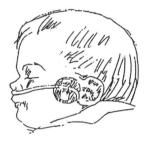

Correct positioning of nasal cannula

VI.   Safety requirements and precautions

A.   All caregivers should be certified in cardiopulmonary resuscitation (CPR) and first aid.

B.   The child using oxygen should have a health care plan outlining the steps to take in case of emergency.

C.   Caregivers should be able to recognize symptoms of insufficient oxygen in the child and to take appropriate action.

D.   Although oxygen is nonflammable, it can cause fire already ignited to burn faster, so tanks should be kept away from heat or electrical sources, and oxygen tanks should be moved carefully so valves do not get broken.

E.   An all-purpose fire extinguisher should be readily accessible.

F. All oxygen equipment should be checked regularly.

G. No-smoking guidelines should be enforced strictly.

VII. Special needs of oxygen-dependent infants and toddlers

A. Encourage normal activities. Children who use oxygen need to be talked to and played with in the same way as other children.

B. Protect the child from becoming entangled in tubing when learning to crawl or walk.

C. Provide additional stimulation to compensate for any developmental delays.

D. Be aware that children who are oxygen-dependent are more susceptible to respiratory infections; avoid unnecessary exposure.

BIBLIOGRAPHY

Ellmyer P., & Thomas, N. (January, 1982). A guide to your patient's safe home use of oxygen. *Nursing '82,* 56-57.

Flenley, D. C. (1985). Long-term oxygen therapy. *Chest, 86*(1), 99-103.

TRACHEOSTOMY CARE

Objectives:

- Identify basic anatomy of the respiratory tract.
- Give reasons why a child might have a tracheostomy.
- Identify important considerations for the child with a tracheostomy.

I. Who requires a tracheostomy?

    A.   A child born with an abnormal airway (windpipe)

    B.   A child who has a neurological problem that makes breathing difficult

    C.   A child who developed an infection that blocks the windpipe

II. What is a tracheostomy?

    A.   A surgeon makes an opening into the windpipe (the trachea) and puts in a tube to keep it open.

    B.   After the tracheostomy, the child no longer breathes through the nose and mouth but, instead, breathes through the trach tube.

    C.   The child may not be able to make sounds at first because most air no longer passes through the vocal chords.

    D.   The ability to eat usually is not affected.

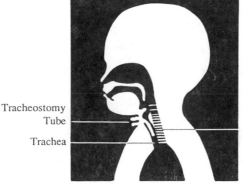

Tracheostomy

III. Important considerations for a child with a tracheostomy

A. Caring for the child with a tracheostomy involves performing invasive procedures. A licensed health care provider such as a registered nurse must care for the child or must provide training and supervision for an individual who is not a licensed health care provider according to state rules and regulations.

B. The child with a tracheostomy should have a health care plan that outlines the possible problems and emergency care that may be needed.

C. If the tracheostomy becomes blocked or falls out:

1. Understand and be able to perform routine procedures for removing obstructions from the trach tube, such as suctioning or changing the trach tube. Only individuals who have been trained and are supervised by a licensed health provider should perform suctioning or change a tracheostomy tube.

2. Be familiar with common problems that may occur with the tracheostomy tube and know:

a. which problems you can handle safely yourself,
b. when to call the nurse consultant or parent/ guardian, and
c. when to call for emergency help.

3. If the tracheostomy or the child's lungs become infected:

a. Recognize the signs of infection.
b. Contact the appropriate person.

D. Illness

1. Children with a trach are more prone to respiratory infections.

2. Vomiting may be a problem, as vomit may get into the trach and cause choking or block the trach tube.

E.   Emergency care

     1.   All adults who care for a child with a trach should know cardiopulmonary resuscitation (CPR). *Breaths are given through the trach tube, not through the nose and mouth.*

     2.   The health care plan should include potential emergency treatment. The plan should address procedures for obtaining emergency care in case of power or telephone failures.

IV.   General care of the child with a tracheostomy

A.   Communication

     1.   Become familiar with the child's alternative communication methods, because the child cannot call out for help.

     2.   Talk to the child as you see and do things together each day to assist learning language and communication.

B.   Have the child wear clothing that will not block the trach tube.

C.   Feeding: Find out from the parent/guardian and the child's doctor

     1.   whether the child can eat safely, and

     2.   what foods are recommended.

D.   Play

     1.   Keep the child with a trach away from water.

     2.   Be sure the child avoids contact sports and sandboxes.

     3.   Be aware that environmental irritants such as pets and wind can cause reactions in the child with a trach.

     4.   Take along appropriate emergency supplies on trips or walks.

BIBLIOGRAPHY

Hazinski, M. F. (1986). Pediatric home tracheostomy care: A parent's guide. *Pediatric Nursing, 12*(1), 41-69.

Kun, S., Halvorson, M., & Liebhauser, P. (1987). *Tracheostomy home care for children.* Los Angeles: Department of Nursing/Children's Hospital of Los Angeles.

Runton, N. (1992). Suctioning artificial airways in children: Appropriate technique. *Pediatric Nursing, 18*(2), 115-118.

Sherman, L. P., & Rosen, C. D. (1990). Development of a preschool program for tracheostomy dependent children. *Pediatric Nursing, 16*(4), 357-361.

Turnage, C. S., & Engleman, S. (1994). Discharge education for parents of infants with tracheostomies. *Journal of Pediatric Nursing, 9(6)*, 425-426.

GASTROSTOMY CARE

Objectives:

- Observe gastrostomy tube feeding and recognize why it is necessary for some children.

- Recognize important factors to consider when caring for a child who requires a gastrostomy tube feeding.

I. Who requires a gastrostomy?

A. Children born with abnormalities of the throat, stomach, or intestines that make it impossible to eat normally.

B. Children who have neurological problems that make sucking and swallowing difficult.

C. Some tiny premature infants who are too weak to suck.

D. Children who have a respiratory problem, a problem with metabolism, or a disease that makes it hard for them to eat enough to grow.

E. Children who need a gastrostomy to "burp."

II. What is gastrostomy feeding?

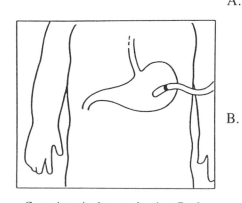

Gastrointestinal tract showing G-tube

A. When a child cannot eat or cannot get enough fluids or nutrition by mouth, a medical specialist makes an opening through the wall of the abdomen into the stomach.

B. The purpose of a gastrostomy is to make sure the child has enough nutrition to grow and be healthy. Some children need a gastrostomy for only a short time, some for much longer.

III. Types of gastrostomies and tubes

A. Gastrostomies, or openings into the stomach, are of two different types, each requiring a different type of feeding tube, feeding procedure, and method of replacing the tube.

1. A tube (called a G-tube) is kept in place in the stomach at all times.

2. The wall of the stomach is used to make a kind of permanent tunnel into which a catheter is inserted at intervals for feeding.

B. Types of gastrostomy tubes

   1. Straight tubes with ends that expand to keep tube from coming out

   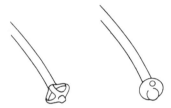

   Examples of straight tubes

   2. Balloon-type tubes and Foley tube, the end of which is inflated with water after insertion to keep it from coming out

   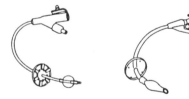

   Examples of balloon-type tubes   *Foley tube*

   3. Skin-level feeding device, which lies flat on the stomach

   Examples of skin-level feeding devices

C.   The child's physician decides which type of tube to use.

D.   Each type of tube has a slightly different procedure for feeding.

IV. Important considerations for tube feeding

A.   Gastrostomy tube feeding is an invasive procedure. A licensed health care provider, such as a nurse, should perform the tube feeding, or should provide training and supervision for the caregiver in a childcare or preschool setting.

B.   In most states a physician's prescription is required for tube feeding in childcare or preschool settings.

C.   The caregiver should understand the procedure the child's family uses at home for the tube feeding, including

    1.   what type of gastrostomy tube the child has,

    2.   what type of formula is used, and how much,

    3.   how fast the tube feeding should be given,

    4.   how much water should be given with the formula,

    5.   when the tube feeding should be given, and

    6.   if the child is allowed to eat food by mouth as well.

D.   The child with gastrostomy tube feeding should have a health care plan that outlines the possible problems and emergency care that may be required.

E.   Caregivers should be familiar with common problems that may occur during tube feeding and recognize

    1.   which problems they can safely handle themselves,

    2.   when to call the nurse or the parent/guardian for help, and

    3.   when to call for emergency help.

F.   Caregivers should be certified in first aid and in cardiopulmonary resuscitation (CPR).

G. Caregivers should follow proper handwashing procedures and wear gloves when giving tube feeding.

V. Daily activities

A. Consider children with G-tubes as a lot more like other children than unlike them.

B. Include the child with a G-tube in the other children's activities.

C. Have the child with a G-tube sit at the table with the other children for meals and snacks.

D. Include all children in the circle of friends. All children need to be touched, talked to, played with, read to.

BIBLIOGRAPHY

Paarlberg, J., & Balint, J. P. (1985). Gastrostomy tubes: Practical guidelines for home care. *Pediatric Nursing, 11*(2), 99-102.

GLOSSARY

GLOSSARY

NOTE: The glossary defines terms as they are used in this *Handbook*. The terms may have other meanings in different contexts.

ABC check: a first aid survey of conditions threatening the life of an accident victim, including checking the *a*irway (for obstruction), *b*reathing, and *c*irculation (checking for a pulse and severe bleeding).

Abduction: the movements of arm and/or leg muscles away from the body.

Abduction wedge: an adaptive device used to keep the legs apart.

Abnormal: not normal; irregular.

Abrasion: a scraping away of a portion of the surface of the skin.

Absence seizure (petit mal): a seizure disorder characterized by a "staring spell," common in children (ages 5-15 years) that usually lasts seconds but may occur frequently (100 times a day).

Acyanotic (Pink) baby: a child whose skin coloring is not affected and looks normal even though a heart defect is present.

ADA: *see Americans with Disabilities Act.*

Adaptability: the ease at which a person adapts to new situations; a component of temperament.

Adaptive: able to adjust to a new use; promoting healthy adjustment.

Adaptive equipment: any assistive device, commercial or homemade, used to maximize ability to function and minimize efforts needed to interact with one's environment.

Adaptive skills: competencies required to meet the daily demands of diverse community settings.

Adduction: the movements of arm and/or leg muscles toward the body.

Adventitious: acquired (not congenital).

AFO: *see Ankle-Foot Orthosis.*

Airborne: traveling through the air.

Allergen: a substance that may provoke an allergic reaction, such as animal dander, dust mites, molds, pollens, and certain foods, medications.

Altruism: acting unselfishly to help someone else.

Amblyopia (Lazy eye): a condition in which one eye is not being used.

American Sign Language (ASL or Ameslan): a gestural form of communication that has most of the features of spoken English.

Americans with Disabilities Act (ADA): the federal civil rights legislation enacted in 1991, prohibiting discrimination against people with disabilities and requiring all public and commercial facilities to make *reasonable accommodations* to allow people with disabilities to use those facilities.

Ameslan: *see American Sign Language.*

Amino acids: substances involved in building new tissue, hormones, enzymes, and antibodies.

Anal: pertaining to the anus.

Ankle-Foot Orthosis (AFO): a splint or brace from the knee to the foot that may have a movable ankle joint; used to correct ankle/foot position and movement.

Antibiotics: a class of medications used to treat non-viral infections.

Anticonvulsant: a medication used to prevent or stop seizures.

Antiepileptic medication: a medication prescribed to control seizure disorders.

Anti-inflammatory drugs: a group of medications that reduce swelling inside the airways and may be taken by inhalation, syrup, or tablets.

Anus: the outer opening of the bowel through which feces are excreted.

Apathy: indifference, lack of interest.

Apnea: a condition characterized by cessation of breathing for 20 seconds or longer or shorter episodes associated with bradycardia, cyanosis, or pallor.

Apnea/bradycardia monitor: a mechanical device that sounds an alarm if infant stops breathing or heart rate drops below a set rate; slow heartbeat monitor.

Apnea monitor: a mechanical device that documents stoppages of breathing in infants.

Approach-withdrawal: the tendency to consistently go near or consistently avoid new situations, people, places, or objects; a component of temperament.

Artificial respiration: a mechanical or other method of breathing for a person who is otherwise unable to breathe.

ASL: *see American Sign Language.*

Assessment: evaluation, appraisal.

Asthma: a chronic lung disease characterized by swelling of the lining of airways that blocks or narrows the airways causing less air flow.

Astigmatism: a common eye condition that results in blurred vision; correctable with prescription lenses.

Asymptomatic: without symptoms.

Ataxic cerebral palsy: a condition characterized by irregular muscle action and lack of muscle coordination, broad-based, lurching gait and problems with balance.

Athetoid cerebral palsy: *see Dyskinetic cerebral palsy.*

Atlantoaxial: pertaining to the first two vertebrae in the neck.

Atonic: lacking normal muscle tone or strength.

Atonic seizures (Drop attacks): a seizure disorder occurring in children (infant through school-age) in which the child suddenly collapses and falls (infant may slump over). Within 10 seconds to 1 minute, the child regains consciousness.

Attachment: an enduring emotional bond between infant and mother developing out of countless hours of interaction.

Attention span: the amount of time a person remains engaged in an activity; a component of temperament.

Attitude: a representation of values and beliefs; consisting of knowledge, feelings, and actions toward an individual, group, or subject.

Atypical: not typical, abnormal, unusual.

Audiogram: a chart produced during a hearing test that shows how well a person can hear different sounds.

Audiologists: a professional who is master's- or doctorally-educated in the study of hearing.

Audiometry: the use of an electrical instrument that measures the softest individual tones and speech sounds an individual can hear and the clarity of what he/she hears.

Auditory: pertaining to the sense of hearing.

Auditory impairment: an inability to hear or process sounds and speech adequately, which in young children hinders learning to understand and produce speech.

Augmentative forms of communication: alternatives to spoken language including sign language, communication boards or devices.

Aura: a sensation such as a smell, memory, feeling, or sound that occurs just before a seizure.

Autistic: pertaining to autism.

Autism: a condition which impairs the ability to have meaningful contact with the surrounding environment, including the people in it.

Autonomy: the desire to do things independently.

Axillary: the hollow area beneath the arm, armpit.

Axillary crutch: the traditional crutch placed beneath the armpit and reaching to the floor; weight is borne on handrests.

Babinski's reflex: an involuntary response stimulated by stroking the sole of the foot upward from heel on the outer side and across the ball of the foot, causing the big toe to bend up and all toes to fan out; a normal response in infants but not in older children and adults.

Behavior management: a group of strategies to encourage appropriate behavior and address problems in behavior.

Behavior modification: a class of psychological treatments that alter behavior by systematically rewarding desired responses and/or punishing or ignoring undesirable responses.

Benign focal epilepsy: a seizure disorder that appears around age 4-10 and disappears in adolescence; seizures occur during sleep that are characterized by twitching of the face, spreading to other parts of the body.

Bladder: the storage vessel in the body that holds urine.

Body jacket: a plastic-like jacket that fits securely around a child's trunk; to help correct scoliosis (curvature of the spine).

BPD: *see Bronchopulmonary dysplasia.*

Brachial artery: a blood vessel that carries aerated blood away from the heart; located between the elbow and shoulder of the inner arm.

Bradycardia: a heart rate below 80 beats per minute in an infant.

Breach: failure to act toward another as a reasonably prudent person would under the circumstances.

Bronchodilator: a medication that relaxes muscles around airways; may be taken by inhalation, syrup, or capsules.

Bronchopulmonary dysplasia (BPD): a condition characterized by damage to the airways usually resulting from mechanical ventilation used to treat life-threatening acute respiratory illness in premature infants.

Calorie: a unit of measurement of heat content or energy.

Candida: a yeast infection.

Cannula: a small tube (catheter) inserted in the body.

Carbohydrate: a compound of carbon, hydrogen and oxygen found in food, including sugars (simple carbohydrates) from fruits and milk, and starches and fiber (complex carbohydrates).

Carbon dioxide: a gas produced as a waste product, transported by blood to the lungs, and exhaled through the nose and mouth.

Cardiopulmonary resuscitation (CPR): the use of artificial respiration and chest compressions to restore breathing and circulation.

Carotid artery: a blood vessel that carries aerated blood away from the heart and is located in the groove between the windpipe and muscles at the side of the neck.

Cataract: the loss of transparency of the lens of the eye or related structures.

Catheter: a tube inserted into the body to allow passage of fluid (liquid or gas) from or into a body cavity.

Catheterization: *see Clean Intermittent Catheterization.*

Celiac disease: a metabolic disorder causing a allergic-like reaction to gluten (in cereal grains and flour).

Cerebral palsy (CP): a general term referring to a variety of conditions that share an impairment in voluntary muscle control and coordination that results in an inability to maintain normal postures and balance and to perform normal movement and skills; arising from oxygen deprivation or damage to the brain.

Chest compressions: the intermittent pressure on the chest used in cardiopulmonary resuscitation (CPR).

Chest physical therapy (CPT): the process of clapping on (or vibrating) the child's chest in different positions to promote drainage.

Chicken pox: a highly contagious viral disease characterized by a generalized, blistering rash over the body that usually erupts 14-16 days after exposure.

Child Find: the public service that identifies and serves qualified children with disabilities from birth through 5 years of age.

Child-proof: to make the environment safe for a young child; removing dangerous substances or eliminating access to dangerous places.

Chromosome: the material within every body cell that carries genetic information determining the inherited characteristics of an individual.

Chronic illness: a prolonged or even lifelong sickness.

CIC: *see Clean Intermittent Catheterization.*

Clean intermittent catheterization (CIC): an invasive procedure in which a clean rubber or plastic catheter is inserted into the urethra and up into the bladder five or six times a day, using a clean nonsterile technique, to release urine and empty the bladder.

Cleft palate: a deformity in which there is a large space in the roof of the mouth.

Clonic convulsions: a type of seizure in which the muscles tense up and relax in rapid succession.

CMV: *see Cytomegalovirus.*

Cognitive delay (Cognitive disability): a problem with attention, memory, problem solving, and/or concept development.

Coining: a traditional Vietnamese treatment for minor illnesses in which a coin is rubbed over the surface of the skin, causing discoloration.

Colostomy: the surgical creation of an artificial opening to the colon.

Communication: the transmission of a message from one person to another.

Competence: the ability to do things independently.

Complex partial seizure: a type of seizure lasting a few minutes in which the individual appears confused and clumsy, and may wander off; sometimes including post-ictal (following the seizure) confusion.

Compressed gas: a type of oxygen delivery system, using pressure allowing the gas to fit into a smaller space (a tank of manageable size).

Conductive hearing loss: an impairment in which sound is blocked or is not transmitted to the inner ear.

Congenital: present at birth.

Congenital heart defects: incomplete or abnormal development of the heart in utero while in the womb, resulting in deformities of the heart at birth.

Congestive heart failure: a condition in which extra blood flow to the lungs places an extra workload on the heart, causing it to pump less efficiently.

Conjunctivitis (Pink eye): a bacterial or viral infection of the clear membranes of the white part of eye and inside of the eyelid; characterized by very inflamed eyes, tearing, itchiness or burn sensations, with possible sensitivity to light or discharge of pus (especially after sleeping).

Contagious: infectious, "catching."

Contracture: a permanent muscle contraction.

Cortical visual impairment: the brain is unable to receive and interpret visual information but there is no structural abnormality in the eyeball.

CP: *see Cerebral palsy.*

CPR: *see Cardiopulmonary resuscitation.*

Crede method: a manual means of expressing urine from the bladder.

Crib death: *see Sudden Infant Death Syndrome.*

Critical periods: the points in human development when the child is ready physiologically to achieve major developmental milestones in movement and coordination, speech and language, and cognitive development; deprivation of adequate stimulation during these periods creates serious, lasting effects.

Croup: an inflammation of the windpipe (trachea) that results in hoarseness and a barking cough.

Cultural norm: the social standard for acceptable behavior regarding such issues as expression of emotion or feelings, religion, and response to illness, disability, and death.

Cupping: a traditional Vietnamese healing method utilizing a cup or glass to create suction on the skin, causing a bruise.

Cutaway cup: a drinking vessel showing the level of liquid in the cup; minimizes tipping of the head backward while drinking.

Cyanosis: a color change in which the lips, nailbeds, or skin around the eyes may have a bluish hue.

Cyanotic (blue) baby: a child whose unoxygenated or "blue" blood is circulated throughout the body, resulting in a bluish cast to the baby's skin.

Cystic fibrosis (CF): a genetic disease affecting the exocrine (mucus-producing) glands in which secretions of thick mucus prevent normal functioning of body organs (most commonly, lungs, digestive system, and sweat glands).

Cytomegalovirus (CMV): a common viral infection among children ages 1-3 that can be transmitted by direct contact with body fluids (saliva, urine, feces), characterized by few or no symptoms among children but poses risk of severe defects to fetuses of pregnant women who are not immune.

Dehydration: the excessive loss of body fluids.

Delay of gratification: postponement of rewarding oneself.

Denis Brown splint: usually two shoes attached to a metal bar to separate and place the feet in proper position; used to correct club feet.

Dental caries: tooth decay occurring when certain bacteria cause teeth to become infected and to demineralize, usually appearing as white chalky areas, or brown spots or craters.

Dental plaque: an accumulation of oral microorganisms and their products that firmly attaches to teeth.

Development: the natural progression from a less complex to a more complex stage, including the biologic, intellectual, behavioral, and social skills domains.

Developmental checklist: an instrument used to assess or describe a child's progress in several areas (such as cognitive development, language development, motor development, and social development) according to the usual *sequence* of development.

Developmental delay: a level of physical, cognitive, adaptive, emotional, or social functioning that is less than expected for a child's age.

Developmental milestones: the achievement of specific skills and abilities (such as an infant's ability to turn over, first steps, or stages of language acquisition) and the passage through major life events (such as sexual maturation, childbearing, menopause) that usually occur in a set order.

Diabetes mellitus (Juvenile diabetes): a metabolic disease characterized by inability of the pancreas to produce insulin; requires daily insulin injection.

Diagnosis: the determination of the nature of an illness or disability.

Diarrheal gastrointestinal disease: an illness caused by viruses or other agents that is spread by fecal-oral contamination; characterized by an increase in the frequency, amount, and liquid content of bowel movements; may be accompanied by nausea and vomiting.

Diplegia: the paralysis of corresponding parts on both sides of the body.

Disability: a physical or mental impairment which substantially limits one or more of the major life activities such as caring for oneself, performing manual tasks, walking, seeing, hearing, speaking, breathing, learning and working (as defined by the Americans with Disabilities Act).

Disability-blind: the ability to focus on the person rather than the person's disability.

Dislocated hips: a condition in which the hip bone has moved out of its socket; can be present at birth.

Distractibility: the ease or difficulty with which a person is interrupted while engaged in an activity; a component of temperament.

Diversity: the existence of differences among people in ethnicity, culture, religion, language, socioeconomic status, and presence or absence of a disability or chronic condition.

Down syndrome: a common genetic disorder in which the child is born with an extra chromosome or extra part of a chromosome (21st pair) resulting in mild to severe mental retardation.

DPT: a vaccine given in a series beginning at 2 months of age to immunize children against diphtheria, tetanus, and pertussis.

Drop attacks: *see Atonic seizures.*

Dust mites: microscopic animals that live in dust, especially in mattresses and overstuffed furniture.

Duty: the obligation to act toward another as a reasonably prudent person would under the circumstances.

Dysfunction: difficult or abnormal functioning.

Dyskinetic cerebral palsy (Athetoid cerebral palsy): a form of cerebral palsy; characterized by slow, wormlike, writhing, involuntary movements that usually are aggravated by stress and absent during sleep.

Ear, Nose, and Throat physician (ENT): a medical doctor with specialized training in the evaluation and medical and surgical treatment of the ears, nose, and throat (formerly called otolaryngologist or otologist).

Early and Periodic Screening, Diagnosis and Treatment Program (EPSDT): a federal funding program for medical services necessary to maintain improved functioning level, developmental or health status of children from birth through 21 years.

Early intervention: the recognition, diagnosis, and treatment of developmental delay or potential delay in children birth to 5 years old; including infant stimulation, therapy, family support and education, specialized health services, and coordination of services.

Emaciated: an excessively thin, wasted condition of the body.

Emergency Medical System (EMS): the public system of response and treatment for medical or other health emergencies; often accessed by dialing 911 on the telephone.

Emotional neglect: lack of attention and love.

Empathy: the ability to experience the thoughts and feelings of another person; understanding another person's feelings and responses.

EMS: Emergency Medical System.

Encephalitis: an inflammation of the brain.

Encopresis: the failure to hold bowel movements for elimination at the proper place.

ENT: *see Ear, Nose, and Throat physician.*

Environmental print: stimuli that maximize reading opportunities by labeling play areas, using menus, and posting simple signs.

Enzyme: a substance that speeds up a chemical change, particularly in the digestion of foods.

Epiglottis: the lid-like tissue that covers the windpipe when swallowing.

Epiglottitis: a rapidly developing bacterial infection, requiring urgent emergency care; causes swelling of epiglottis that may block the airway; characterized by apprehension, drooling, and difficulty swallowing, speaking, and breathing.

Epilepsy: a chronic condition characterized by repeated, unprovoked seizures.

Episodic: occurring at intervals.

Expectorant: a medication to treat respiratory infections by encouraging the coughing up of mucus.

Extension: movements that straighten the arms or legs.

Extensor hypertonicity: arching of the back.

Extinction: the elimination (disappearance) of a behavior that receives no response.

Extremities: the limbs (arms and legs).

Failure to thrive: a group of symptoms in infants and children who do not gain weight properly; may be organic (caused by disease) or non-organic (caused by neglect, abuse, or improper feeding).

Family: any group of individuals who define themselves as a family and take on the culturally recognized obligations and responsibilities of a family.

Family dynamics: the influence of members of a family upon each other.

Farsightedness: *see Hyperopia.*

Fats: a component of foods found in vegetable oils, animal fats, dairy products, and breast milk, necessary for growth, healthy skin, and insulation against heat loss.

Febrile seizure: a type of seizure that occurs during a fever; characterized by generalized, convulsive-type movements of the body.

Fecal: pertaining to feces.

Feces: bowel movements.

Fetal alcohol syndrome (FAS): a medical diagnosis made when there is prenatal or postnatal growth retardation (affecting weight, length, and head circumference), a characteristic pattern of facial features *and* central nervous system damage with resulting neurologic abnormalities, developmental delay, or intellectual impairment.

Fetus: the unborn baby.

First-degree burn: a burn characterized by red skin, mild swelling, and pain.

Fisted hand: the position of the hand in which the fingers are doubled up into the palm.

Flammable: able to be burnt, combustible.

Flexion: bending.

Floor stander: an adaptive device that provides support while standing.

Floppy baby: an infant with low muscle tone at birth.

FO: *see Foot Orthosis.*

Focal seizure (Partial seizure): a sudden, unusual discharge of electrical energy in a limited part of the brain.

Fontanel: the soft spot in an infant's head.

Foot Orthosis (FO): a heel cup or foot support, or both; used to correct heel or foot position.

Full-term infant: an infant born at 40 weeks of gestational age (40 weeks after conception).

Fungal diaper rash: an irritation caused by a fungus and characterized by a red area on the buttocks surrounded by raw-looking areas.

G-tube: *see Gastrostomy tube.*

Gastroesophageal reflux: in infants, a non-seizure condition that produces frequent vomiting but looks like a "convulsion."

Gastroesophageal reflux: regurgitation of stomach contents into the esophagus.

Gastrostomy: a surgically created opening through the wall of the abdomen into the stomach constructed when a child cannot eat or cannot get enough fluids or nutrition by mouth.

Gastrostomy tube (G-tube): a tube device inserted into the stomach through a surgically created opening for the purpose of directly conveying nutrients to the stomach.

Generalized seizure: a sudden, unusual discharge of electrical energy involving most of the brain.

Generalized tonic-clonic seizure (Grand mal): a type of seizure; characterized by loss of consciousness, stiffening and shaking of entire body, and possibly pallor or bluish color around the mouth; lasts 2 to 15 minutes (usually less than 5) and is followed by a post-ictal state (confusion).

Genetic: inherited; pertaining to heredity.

Genitals (Genitalia): the external sex organs.

German measles: *see Rubella.*

Gestational age: age since conception, rather than birth.

Gesture: a non-verbal signal.

Gingivitis: an inflammation, redness, and puffiness of the gums.

Grand mal: *see Generalized tonic-clonic seizure.*

Grimace: a distortion of the face.

Gross motor: pertaining to the large muscles of the body, such as those used for walking or throwing.

Growth: the increase in size of all or part of a living being in the process of development.

Gustatory: pertaining to the sense of taste.

H flu: *see Haemophilus influenza type B.*

Habilitation: the acquisition of new skills to reach age-appropriate developmental milestones.

Haemophilus influenza type B: a bacteria responsible for illnesses including meningitis and epiglottitis.

Handicap: a limitation in functioning as a consequence of a disability.

Handling: assisting a person to move using specific holding positions or movements.

Hard measles: *see Rubeola.*

HAV: *see Hepatitis.*

HBV: *see Hepatitis.*

Head lice: a parasitic infestation caused by lice detectable when nits (white lice eggs) are seen attached to the hair shaft and resulting in itchiness of the scalp.

Head Start: a federally funded program serving children living in low-income areas. At least 10% of all enrollment is reserved for children with disabilities or developmental delays.

Hemiplegia: paralysis involving one side of the body.

Hemisphere: a half of the brain.

Hepatitis: easily spread viral infections causing inflammation of the liver; Hepatitis A (HAV), spread via fecal-oral contamination and characterized by mild flu-like symptoms in young children; Hepatitis B (HBV), usually sexually transmitted and characterized by flu-like symptoms.

Herpes simplex: a viral infection; characterized by a blisterlike sore on mucous membranes that weep clear fluid and slowly crust over.

Herpetic lesion: a cold sore.

Hip-Knee-Ankle-Foot Orthosis (HKAFO): a splint or brace connected by a pelvic band around the lower back; used to control position and movement of hips, knees, ankles, and feet.

HIV: *see Human Immunodeficiency Virus.*

HIV antibodies: the protective substances the body produces to combat the HIV virus.

HKAFO: *see Hip-Knee-Ankle-Foot Orthosis.*

Holophrase: a single word or sound used to express a more complete phrase (for example, me for I want to do it); occurs early in language development.

Home cardiac/respiratory monitor: a mechanical device that detects breathing or heart rate, or both.

Human Immunodeficiency Virus (HIV): the infectious agent that causes AIDS.

Hydrocephalus: a condition in which fluid in the brain is not absorbed properly; also known as water on the brain.

Hyperopia (farsightedness): a condition in which objects that are far away are seen best; close objects are hard to see.

Hyperplasia: an increase in the number of cells (non-tumorous) in a tissue or organ that increases its bulk.

Hypotonic: having low muscle tone; floppiness.

Hypertonicity: a condition characterized by high muscle tone or rigidity; also called spasticity.

Hypoxic spell: an episode in which a child with a congenital heart defect becomes much bluer or grayish in color, very short of breath, and very limp; may pass out.

IDEA: *see Individuals with Disabilities Education Act.*

IEP: *see Individualized Education Program.*

IFSP: *see Individualized Family Service Plan.*

Impedance monitor: a mechanical device that measures heart rate and respiratory effort (breathing).

Impetigo: a bacterial skin infection characterized by a skin rash with a brownish-yellow (honey colored) crust; often seen around the nose and mouth that may spread to other parts of the body by direct contact.

In utero: within the uterus (womb).

Incidence: the frequency of new cases appearing in a population.

Inclusion: the full integration of children with disabilities into the same settings available to children without disabilities, sharing the same classroom and activities for the entire day.

Incontinence: lack of control; usually pertaining to inability to control urine or bowel movements.

Indian sitting: *see Tailor sitting.*

Individualized Education Program (IEP): a document called for in Part B of IDEA (the Individuals with Disabilities Education Act); prepared for an individual child to describe unique needs, educational and related services required to meet the needs, goals and objectives, assessment methods, and schedules of services.

Individualized Family Service Plan (IFSP): a document derived from Part C of IDEA (the Individuals with Disabilities Education Act); describes early intervention services for an infant or toddler and the child's family; including family support, the child's educational, therapeutic, and health needs.

Individuals with Disabilities Education Act (IDEA): federal legislation that requires each participating state to organize an Interagency Coordinating Council (ICC) and to select a lead agency responsible for ensuring the identification and service planning for children, ages birth to 21 who have or are at risk for developmental disabilities; Part C addresses the needs of children, birth to 3 years of age; Part B addresses children age 3 and older.

Indwelling catheter: a draining tube left in place in the bladder.

Infantile spasms: a syndrome of symptoms occurring in infants 3-12 months of age; includes seizures that tend to occur in clusters and may appear as a nod of the head or a total body jerk (a "jackknife" movement); associated with developmental delays.

Infectious disease: a contagious illness (can be spread from person to person).

Inhibitory cast: a plaster or synthetic cast used to decrease lower extremity extensor tone for better standing and walking.

Intervention: a treatment to correct or alleviate a condition.

Intracranial hemorrhage: bleeding within the brain.

Invasive health care procedure: prescribed physical care that involves penetration of the body (such as injections, oral administration of medicine, G-tube feeding, and catheterization).

Irritable bladder: *see Spastic bladder.*

KAFO: *see Knee-Ankle-Foot Orthosis.*

Kenny sticks: crutches that have bands going around the forearms.

Ketogenic diet: a special diet that may be used to control seizures in certain individuals.

Kidneys: a pair of organs that remove waste products from the blood and produce urine.

Kinesthetic: the muscle sense in which a person knows where his or her body is in relation to the environment.

Knee-Ankle-Foot Orthosis (KAFO): a splint or brace running from above the knee down to the foot; used to control knee/ankle/foot position and movement.

Labeling: the process of referring to a person by emphasizing a disability; putting the disability before the person (for example, a mentally retarded child rather than a child with mental retardation).

Laceration: a wound resulting from the tearing of the skin.

Language: an organized system of symbols people use to communicate with one another.

Lazy eye: *see Amblyopia.*

Learning: the unfolding of genetic programming, or experiences in the environment, or the interaction of genetics and the environment, promoting development of the cognitive, language, motor, social, and emotional domains.

Least restrictive environment (LRE): a concept promoting participation in general education classrooms as the most desirable setting for children with disabilities; intended to decrease the number of children in institutional settings and segregated classrooms.

Legally blind: the condition of having visual acuity less than 20/200 in the better eye with best possible correction; or restriction of the visual field to 20° or less from the normal 180° in the better eye.

Lenox-Gastaut syndrome: a condition that starts in early childhood (ages 1-5 years) involving various types of seizures; associated with mental retardation and developmental delay.

Lesion: a wound or injury.

Liability: the responsibility one bears for the breach of a duty.

Lice: a parasitic insect that can be found in the hair or body of infected humans.

Linguistic: pertaining to language.

Liquid oxygen: a type of oxygen delivery system in which oxygen is cooled to a liquid state for storage in a tank.

Locomotor: pertaining to locomotion, or movement.

Low vision (Partially sighted): the condition of having some functional vision; ranging reliance on vision for learning to relying primarily on hearing, touch, and other senses for learning.

Maladaptive: inappropriate or inadequate.

Mandated reporter: an individual identified by law as required to report suspected or known child abuse or neglect.

Mattress monitor: a mechanical device that measures simple chest wall movements.

Maturation: the achievement of full growth or development.

Measles: *see Rubella; Rubeola.*

Meninges: the membranes surrounding the brain and spinal cord.

Meningitis: a serious bacterial infection that inflames the membranes surrounding the brain or spinal cord; characterized by stiff neck, vomiting, irritability, lcthargy (listlessness); requires immediate medical attention.

Meningocele: a sac protruding out of the spinal column or skull due to a defect in the bones.

Mental retardation: a medical diagnosis referring to substantial limitation in a person's functioning; manifested before age 18; includes intellectual functioning well below average and related limitations in two or more adaptive skills areas.

Metabolism: the process by which an organism ingests, digests, transports, utilizes, and excretes food substances.

Mid-line: the vertical center line in the body.

Migraine: a condition characterized by vomiting, nausea, diarrhea, flushing, or pallor; intolerance to light; confusion; a headache may or may not be present.

Mineral: a non-organic material, usually originating in the earth's crust; required for normal metabolism.

Mixed hearing loss: a combination of conductive and sensorineural hearing loss.

Moro reflex: an inborn, involuntary response evoked by sudden jarring or "drop" in elevation of an infant; causes flaring of the arms and legs and fanning of the fingers with thumb and index finger forming a "c" shape, followed by pulling the arms in to a fetal position, with possible crying.

Motor: pertaining to muscles and their movements.

Motor system: the group of muscles and nerves that produce movements of the body.

Multisensory activities: those that involve speech, hearing, movement, touch, and sight.

Mumps: an infectious disease causing swelling of the salivary glands, and possibly other glands.

Muscle tone: the amount of tension in a muscle or group of muscles.

Myoclonic seizure: a type of seizure appearing in infancy through adolescence; characterized by sudden, brief muscle jerks involving all or part of the body; usually associated with other neurologic problems and developmental delays.

Myopia (Nearsightedness): a condition in which close objects are seen best.

Nasal flaring: the enlargement of the nostrils when one inhales (breathes in).

Natural consequences: the normal or typical results of the child's own actions.

Nearsightedness: *see Myopia.*

Nebulizer: an atomizer, a device for spraying a liquid.

Negligence: the omission or neglect of reasonable precaution, care, or action.

Neurogenic bladder: a condition characterized by loss of voluntary control of the bladder.

Neurogenic bowel: a condition characterized by weakness or loss of voluntary control of rectal sphincter causing constipation, diarrhea, or accidents.

Neurological: pertaining to the nervous system.

Nitrogen: an element vital to the maintenance of existing tissue health.

Nonverbal communication: the passage of information between individuals without the use of words, as by gestures or glances.

Nutrition: the science of food, the nutrients they contain, their action, interaction, and balance in relation to health and disease, and the process of metabolism.

Nystagmus: an involuntary, rapid movement of the eyes.

Oculomotor problem: a condition characterized by uncoordinated eye muscle movements.

Olfactory: referring to the sense of smell.

Ophthalmologist: a physician who diagnoses and treats eye diseases, can perform surgery, and prescribe eyeglasses and medication.

Optic nerve: the nerve that goes from the retina at the back of the eyeball to the back of the brain.

Optic nerve hypoplasia: the congenital underdevelopment of retinal nerve cells; may result in marked visual impairment.

Optometrist: an eye specialist who can prescribe glasses, perform low-vision exams, and may be able to provide some vision training therapy with a vision therapist (for problems such as lazy eye).

Oral thrush: a fungus infection of the mouth.

Orthopedics: the medical specialty dealing with the musculoskeletal system, extremities, and spine.

Orthosis: a brace; custom-made adaptive equipment.

Otitis media: a recurrent infection of the middle ear; often occurs in conjunction with an upper respiratory infection.

Otolaryngologist: *see Ear, Nose, and Throat physician.*

Otologist: *see Ear, Nose, and Throat physician.*

Ototoxic: having a toxic action upon the ear.

Overpraising: overreacting to minor achievements.

Oxygen: a tasteless, odorless gas inhaled into the lungs, passed to the blood, and distributed to vital organs and tissues.

Oxygen therapy: a treatment in which extra oxygen is provided to someone who has breathing difficulties.

Pacemaker: a surgically implanted device that maintains an adequate heart rate.

Palate: the roof of the mouth; separates the mouth from the nasal passages.

Palliative: relieving discomfort from a condition without curing it.

Pallor: paleness.

Palmar grasp: an infant's reflexive reaction elicited by touching the palm of the hand near the base of fingers, causing the fist to clench.

Parapodium: an adaptive device to provide support while standing.

Parasite: a plant or animal that lives on or in another organism.

Part B: *see Individuals with Disabilities Education Act.*

Part C: *see Individuals with Disabilities Education Act.*

Partial seizure: *see Focal seizure.*

Partially sighted: *see Low vision.*

Patronizing: "talking down" to a person.

Pavlic harness: a cloth positioning device with a harness over the chest; used to keep the legs apart to correct hip dislocations.

Peak flow meter: an instrument used to measure air flow in children 4 years and older.

Pediatric HIV infection: human immunodeficiency virus (HIV) infection occurring in children under the age of 13 years; differs from HIV infection in adults in terms of symptoms and the speed with which the disease progresses.

Pelvis: the part of the skeleton that forms a bony girdle at the base of the trunk.

People-first language: a style of expression intended to emphasize a person's humanity over a disability; literally places the person before the disability (such as a *child with a disability*, instead of a *disabled child*).

Perineal: pertaining to the area between the legs from the genital organs to the anus.

Periodic breathing: a normal fluctuation in infant breathing patterns in which breathing stops for 5-10 seconds but spontaneously begins again.

Peripheral vision: the extent of vision to the sides of the area on which the eyes are focused.

Pertussis: a serious, contagious bacterial infection; characterized by a "whoop" sound on inhalation, with coughing spasms.

Petit mal: *see Absence seizure.*

Phenylketonuria (PKU): a metabolic disorder; characterized by the absence of the enzyme needed to break down a specific amino acid in protein (found in infant formulas and dairy products); may lead to development of severe retardation, hyperactivity, and seizures.

Physical abuse: an act of bodily harm inflicted intentionally.

Physical neglect: the failure of the caregiver to provide adequate food, clothing shelter, medical care, or supervision.

Physical therapy: a method of treatment involving the use of heat, cold, light, water, or mechanical apparatus.

Pink baby: *see Acyanotic baby.*

Pink eye: *see Conjunctivitis.*

PKU: *see Phenylketonuria.*

Plantar grasp: a infant's reflexive reaction evoked by touching the soles of the feet near the base of the toes, causing the toes to curl under.

Plasticity: adaptability, flexibility.

Pneumonia: a potentially serious lung infection caused by viruses or bacteria; usually characterized by increased respiratory rate, retractions, grunting, and nasal flaring, with possible fever, chills, chest pain, nausea, vomiting; more likely to occur following an upper respiratory infection.

Poison control center: a place that provides emergency information about poisons, their antidotes, and treatment of individuals who have been poisoned.

Polydrug abuse: the use of multiple drugs, or drugs in combination with alcohol or other central nervous system depressants.

Positioning: physical placement techniques that encourage a person's best functioning.

Post-ictal state: a period after a seizure when the individual is sleepy, lethargic, or not himself/herself.

Posterior walker: a metal frame supporting the person from behind, with wheels on the front; to assist walking.

Poverty: the condition of living with insufficient economic resources; implies material hardship and differentiating experiences (such as preoccupation with survival-related issues).

Poverty line: the federally determined cash income level that defines the condition of being poor; used to determine eligibility for public assistance programs.

Prematurity: the condition of an infant born before full development (nine months).

Preoperational stage: a period of cognitive development lasting from age 2 to age 7 during which a child learns language; proposed by Piaget.

Pressure sores: open sores that form from unrelieved pressure on the skin, including pressure from braces or adaptive equipment.

Prevalence: the number of existing cases of a condition or illness.

Prodrome: a feeling of fear or anxiety that occurs days or hours before a seizure.

Prone: the position of lying on one's stomach.

Prone stander: an adaptive device to provide support to enable standing (may have wheels).

Prosthesis: a replacement for damaged or missing parts; an artificial limb (arm, leg).

Protein: a substance found in food (especially meat, fish, poultry, eggs, and dairy products) that the body breaks down into amino acids and nitrogen.

Psychological maltreatment: negative and hostile verbal and nonverbal treatment.

Psychomotor: relating to the conscious origin of muscle (motor) movement.

Pulse: the expansion and contraction of the heart; can be felt in many places in the body.

Pyramidal cerebral palsy: *see Spastic cerebral palsy.*

Quadriplegia: the involvement of all four extremities.

Reciprocating brace: a hip-knee-ankle-foot orthotic device with an attached cable that moves alternate legs as the wearer shifts weight.

Reciprocity: shared obligation.

Redirection: the replacement of an inappropriate form of an activity or behavior with a more appropriate or acceptable form of the same activity or behavior.

Reflex: involuntary reactions to stimulation that are part of a larger set of fixed behavior patterns; aids in survival, especially in infancy.

Regressive behavior: return to a less mature form of behavior.

Rehabilitation: the restoration of lost functioning.

Reinforcer: a consequence of a behavior that increases (positive reinforcer) or decreases (negative reinforcer) the strength or frequency of the behavior.

Rescue breathing: artificial respiration, or breathing rhythmically into the mouth (and nose of small children) of a person whose natural breathing has stopped.

Retina: the membrane at the back of the inside of the eyeball that receives light waves and transmits them to the brain to produce vision.

Retinopathy: a non-inflammatory degenerative disease of the retina of the eye.

Retractions: the visible pulling of the muscles of the chest in between the ribs; a sign of difficult breathing.

Rhythmicity: the regularity of biological functions such as eating and sleeping; a component of temperament.

Ritual: a routine.

Role reversal: the situation occurring when parties in a relationship assume each other's culturally expected feelings, behaviors, and responsibilities; for example, a child *mothers* the parent.

Rooting: an infant's inborn, involuntary reaction elicited by stroking cheek along side of the mouth, causing an infant to turn toward the side and to begin to suck.

Roseola: a viral infection usually affecting children between ages of 6 months to 36 months; characterized by 3 to 4 days of high fever, followed by a faint, generalized rash, mainly on trunk and back of neck.

Rotary chewing: the action of switching food from side to side within the mouth while keeping the lips closed.

Rubella (Three-day measles): contagious childhood disease with fever, chills, various respiratory symptoms, and rash; lasting about three days; infection of a woman during early pregnancy can cause deformities in the infant.

Rubeola (Hard measles): a highly contagious viral disease; characterized by a fever, cough, and conjunctivitis, followed by generalized rash that is most prominent on face and upper body; can be very severe with many complications; usually lasts about two weeks.

Sacral sitting: an improper posture in which one's weight is shifted back onto the tailbone and the upper back is rounded.

Sacrum: the bone in the spinal column that is between the two hip bones; the tailbone.

Saliva: the liquid secreted into the mouth; spit.

Salivary glands: the glands in the mouth that produce saliva.

Scabies: a parasitic infestation caused by mites that results in itching of the skin, particularly at night; characterized by skin irritation, particularly in skin-fold areas, that may resemble scratches.

Scoliosis: curvature of the spine.

Scotoma: a blind spot in the visual area.

Second-degree burn: a burn characterized by red skin, blistering (open or closed), and severe pain.

Section 504 (of the Rehabilitation Act): the federal civil rights legislation protecting the rights of people with disabilities; schools receiving federal funds must guarantee equal access and equal opportunity to children with and without disabilities.

Segregation: the separation of children with disabilities from children without disabilities; children with disabilities attend special education classes and do not mingle with other children.

Seizure: a sudden, unusual discharge of electrical energy in the brain.

Self-esteem: feelings about self based on the individual's experiences.

Self-regulation: control over one's own behavior.

Sensorimotor: pertaining to both sensory and motor.

Sensorimotor stage: a period of cognitive development lasting from birth to age 18 months during which a child learns about objects and events in environment; proposed by Piaget.

Sensorineural hearing loss: an impairment in which the brain does not understand sound that reaches the inner ear; signals reaching the brain may be loud enough, but are unclear or distorted.

Sensory: pertaining to sensation or the senses.

Separation anxiety: an emotional reaction shown by babies in the second 6 months of life; expressed as uneasiness when parents/guardians leave them, and joyful greeting upon their return.

Sepsis: the presence of organisms that cause disease; infection.

Sex-typed behavior: an interest or activity more typical of one sex than the other.

Sexual abuse: exposure to sexual experiences to which the child cannot consent or that are developmentally inappropriate.

Shaping: the reinforcement of behaviors that are increasingly closer to the desired behavior.

Shock: the condition in which there is inadequate blood flow to the brain, heart, lungs and other vital organs as the body tries to compensate for severe injury.

Short Bowel syndrome: a condition in which a child is unable to digest and absorb nutrients; requires intravenous or gastrointestinal tube feeding to sustain growth.

Shunt: a surgically inserted catheter to drain excess fluid.

Side-lyer: adaptive equipment to assist lying on one's side.

SIDS: *see Sudden Infant Death Syndrome.*

Simple partial seizure: a type of seizure in which the individual may see or feel unusual sensations, turn pale, sweat, flush, or feel sick; jerking motions in one body part progress throughout the body; unusual in young children.

Social deprivation: the lack of environmental stimulation adequate to promote full development.

Spastic bladder (Irritable bladder): a condition of uncontrolled muscle contraction causing intermittent leakage of urine.

Spastic cerebral palsy (Pyramidal cerebral palsy): a condition characterized by hypertonicity (rigidity) of the extremities and hypotonicity (floppiness) of the neck and trunk; also present are persistence of primitive reflexes, poor control of posture, balance, and coordinated movement, resulting joint and bone deformities, and slow, labored movements.

Spasticity: *see Hypertonicity.*

Spatial: pertaining to space.

Speech: production of the sounds of a language when they are organized into words and word groups.

Speech/language pathologist: a professional who is master's- or doctorally-educated in the evaluation of and therapy techniques for speech and language development.

Speech therapy: treatments and exercises to improve verbal sound production and articulation (pronunciation).

Sphincter: a muscle that encircles a duct, tube or orifice (body opening), and contracts or opens.

Spina bifida: a birth defect of the spinal column that results in muscle weakness or paralysis or both, as well as a lack of sensation below the area of the defect.

Splint: a device used to hold broken bones together or to protect a body part and keep it in proper position.

Status epilepticus: a prolonged seizure or series of uncontrolled seizures that continue non-stop for 20 minutes or more.

Stepping: a reflexive reaction occurring when an infant is held erect with the sole of the foot on a hard surface, causing simulated walking movements.

Stereotype: the assumption that all people with a certain characteristic (for example, a disability, racial, religious, ethnic group membership, and so on) are alike.

Stereotypic behavior: the constant repetition of certain meaningless gestures or movements (such as rocking, head rolling, staring at fingers), and other odd, repeated movements.

Strabismus: a condition in which the eyes are crossed or misaligned; the eyes do not focus on the same object at the same time.

Stranger distress: a baby's negative emotional reaction to the presence of an unfamiliar person; typically appears between the ages of 7 and 10 months, lasts 2 to 3 months.

Strep throat: an infection caused by streptococcal bacteria resulting in a very red, sore throat; may be accompanied by coldlike symptoms and fever.

Sudden Infant Death Syndrome (SIDS, Crib death): the abrupt and seemingly unexplained death of a healthy infant.

Supine: lying on one's back.

Suspension: a liquid with particles dispersed in it.

Symbolic play: imaginary or make-believe play; crucial to development of abstract thought.

Symmetry: the state in which two sides are balanced or matching; mirror image.

Syndrome: a group of related symptoms or characteristics of a condition or illness.

Tactile: referring to the sense of touch.

Tailor sitting: sitting with one's knees far apart and legs crossed at the ankle; previously called *Indian sitting*.

Temperament: the inborn, biologically-based individual differences that affect how a child reacts and adjusts to changes in the environment.

Third-degree burn: a burn characterized by red, white or charred skin, and loss of skin layers.

Three-day measles: *see Rubella.*

Threshold of responsiveness: the strength a stimulus must be or achieve to cause a person to respond; a component of temperament.

Thrush: a fungal infection of the mouth; characterized by white patches, resembling milk, that coat the tongue and inside of cheeks but do not rinse out or wipe off.

Title V: the federal legislation that funds programs for children with disabilities of families living below or near the poverty line; usually administered through state health departments; also referred to as "programs for children with special health care needs" or "programs for children with disabilities."

Toddlerhood: the period of transition from infancy to childhood (usually ages 1½ to about 3 years) during which dramatic social, emotional, and cognitive changes occur.

Tone-Reducing Ankle-Foot Orthosis (TRAFO): a splint designed to decrease lower extremity extensor tone; corrects ankle/foot positioning and movement to make standing and walking easier.

Tonic neck reflex: an infant's inborn response when the head is turned to one side and the arm and leg on that side extend while the opposite arm and leg draw toward the body.

Total communication: a communication system for people with auditory impairments that combines an oral and a sign system.

Toxin: a poison.

Trachea: the windpipe.

Tracheostomy: a surgical procedure creating an opening in the windpipe (trachea) into which a tube is inserted so that breathing occurs though the tube rather than the nose and mouth.

Traction: a pulling method for treating broken and dislocated bones.

TRAFO: *see Tone-Reducing Ankle-Foot Orthosis.*

Transition: the movement from one activity, stage, or phase to the next.

Trauma: a severe injury or wound; either physical or psychological.

Trigger: an aspect of the environment that makes asthma symptoms appear or worsen; includes irritants, allergens, strong emotions, and vigorous exercise.

Trunk: the torso; the main part of the body; the shoulders through the hips.

Tunnel vision: a condition in which the visual field is constricted (like looking through a straw).

Tympanometry: the use of an instrument that tests the ear drum and middle ear system to determine proper sound transfer to the inner ear.

Unconscious: unresponsive, unaware.

Ureters: the two muscular tubes that drain urine from the kidneys to the bladder.

Urethra: the muscular tube through which urine flows from the bladder out of the body.

URI: an infection of the upper respiratory tract.

Verbal: pertaining to speaking and language.

Visual acuity: the clarity or sharpness of the image seen.

Visual field: the total area seen.

Visual impairment: the loss of eyesight as a result of damage to the eye itself, the optic nerve along its pathway, or visual centers of the brain.

Vitamin: an organic substance found in food (fruits, vegetables, dairy products, cereals, grains, seeds, beans, oil, meats, and fish); may be either water-soluble (cannot be stored in the body) or fat-soluble (can be stored in the body); vital for normal metabolism.

W-sitting: an improper posture where one's legs are bent out and backward from the knee, spread away from either side of the torso (legs are in the shape of a W).

Water on the brain: *see Hydrocephalus.*

Wedge: an adaptive device used in positioning children.

Wheezing: a high-pitched sound heard upon breathing, in certain respiratory conditions (such as asthma).

Whooping cough: *see Pertussis.*

Working poor: low-income wage earners whose families are above the poverty line but face economic hardship.